UNDERSTANDING LEADERSHIP
LEADERSHIP
for Nursing Associates

Sara Miller McCune founded SAGE Publishing in 1965 to support the dissemination of usable knowledge and educate a global community. SAGE publishes more than 1000 journals and over 800 new books each year, spanning a wide range of subject areas. Our growing selection of library products includes archives, data, case studies and video. SAGE remains majority owned by our founder and after her lifetime will become owned by a charitable trust that secures the company's continued independence.

Los Angeles | London | New Delhi | Singapore | Washington DC | Melbourne

HAZEL COWLS
SARAH TOBIN
NATALIE CUSACK

UNDERSTANDING LEADERSHIP

for Nursing Associates

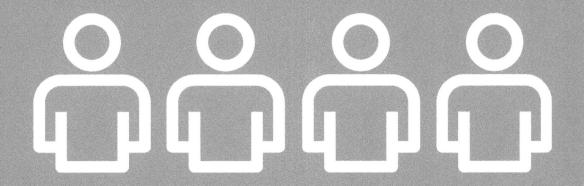

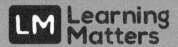

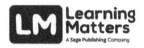

Learning Matters
A Sage Publishing Company
1 Oliver's Yard
55 City Road
London EC1Y 1SP

Sage Publications Inc.
2455 Teller Road
Thousand Oaks, California 91320

Sage Publications India Pvt Ltd
B 1/l 1 Mohan Cooperative Industrial Area
Mathura Road
New Delhi 110 044

Sage Publications Asia-Pacific Pte Ltd
3 Church Street
#10-04 Samsung Hub
Singapore 049483

Editor: Martha Cunneen
Development editor: Lyndsay Oliver/Ruth Lilly
Senior project editor: Chris Marke
Marketing manager: Ruslana Khatagova
Cover design: Wendy Scott
Typeset by: C&M Digitals (P) Ltd, Chennai, India
Printed in the UK

Library of Congress Control Number: 2023941480

British Library Cataloguing in Publication Data

A catalogue record for this book is available
from the British Library

ISBN 978-1-5296-0592-1
ISBN 978-1-5296-0591-4 (pbk)

At Sage we take sustainability seriously. Most of our products are printed in the UK using responsibly
sourced papers and boards. When we print overseas we ensure sustainable papers are used as measured
by the Paper Chain Project grading system. We undertake an annual audit to monitor our sustainability.

Contents

Contents

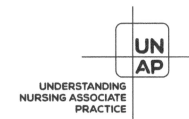

**UNDERSTANDING
NURSING ASSOCIATE
PRACTICE**

Supporting you through your nursing associate training & career

UNDERSTANDING NURSING ASSOCIATE PRACTICE is a series uniquely designed for trainee nursing associates.

Each book in the series is:
- Mapped to the NMC standards of proficiency for nursing associates
- Affordable
- Full of practical activities & case studies
- Focused on clearly explaining theory & its application to practice

Other books in the series include:

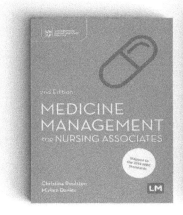

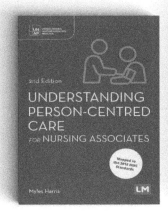

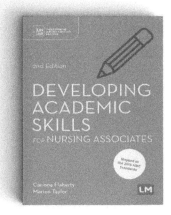

Visit
uk.sagepub.com/UNAP
to see the full collection

Acknowledgements

Thank you to Jenita Loheswaran, who was willing to share her experiences of leadership while studying on the FDNA programme.

About the authors

Hazel Cowls is an NMC registered adult nurse and teacher, a registered non-medical prescriber with a background in cardiac nursing. She is currently a Lecturer in Adult Nursing at the University of Plymouth and teaches leadership and management modules. She has an MSc in Contemporary Healthcare (Education) and is a Fellow of the Higher Education Academy. Hazel has an interest in compassionate leadership and team-working and how this contributes to safe, effective care.

Sarah Tobin is an NMC registered adult nurse, mental health nurse and teacher and has worked in emergency care, elderly care, oncology and cancer screening, as well as gastroenterology. Currently working as a Lecturer in Adult Nursing at the University of Plymouth, she also continues to work as a Clinical Nurse Specialist at Torbay and South Devon NHS Foundation Trust. Sarah's MSc and subsequent PhD research focused on defining compassion in healthcare and how this can be demonstrated. The findings confirmed her belief that compassionate care is a clinically relevant and important skill that all healthcare staff need to demonstrate.

Natalie Cusack is an NMC registered mental health nurse and teacher with a background in working with adults with complex mental health needs. Currently working as a Lecturer of Nursing at University of Plymouth, Natalie has an interest in teaching on the Foundation Degree Nursing Associate programme and digital health.

Introduction

Who is this book for?

This book has been written to help support and inform trainee nursing associates (TNAs) as it makes very direct links to the relevant Nursing and Midwifery Council (NMC) Standards of Proficiency. However, the content is applicable to nurses in any field and at any level of their continuing educational endeavours. Leadership is a key element of all nursing roles which, most crucially, has a direct impact on the effectiveness of patient care. Whatever environment a nurse works in, leadership skills will be transferable and applicable; this book aims to present an interesting and meaningful exploration of different aspects of leadership. As the nursing associate (NA) role becomes more established and embeds into the nursing workforce, the need to understand and practise effectively as a leader also becomes more apparent. Whether a TNA aims to become and remain a registered nursing associate (RNA) or whether they aspire to further development, the need to understand and practise meaningful leadership skills will be vital.

About the book

NAs are in the unique position of being able to practise across all fields of nursing with a single qualification. It is important therefore to maximise those skills that are universal, transferable and applicable – leadership is clearly just such a skill. The NA role was established to 'bridge the gap' between the healthcare assistant and the registered nurse; this may lead one to conclude that leadership would be the preserve of the registered nurse. This book aims to disavow anyone who reads it of that perception, and to firmly establish the idea that leadership is a requirement of the NA, whatever role they undertake.

Each chapter can stand alone and act as a clear and informative resource to help develop your understanding of why leadership is important and all of the many elements of nursing practice and patient care that are impacted by it. However, taken as a whole, the eight chapters form a comprehensive exploration of leadership, leadership theory and leadership practice in relation to the nursing profession and, specifically, the new and ever-developing role of the NA.

The authors have aimed to make the chapters engaging and informative and to challenge you to think about your nursing practice. Understanding the wider structure of healthcare organisations may not seem important initially, but as a nurse you have direct and vital contact with patients – who better to influence the decision-makers? To do that you need to understand how they work. Such understanding and engagement link directly to leadership and, ultimately, to optimising and improving patient care.

The nursing profession is the bedrock of health provision, the largest professional group of healthcare providers by a considerable margin. Challenge, working in pressurised environments and adapting to rapidly changing circumstances are not new concepts for healthcare professionals. The modern era with new technological capabilities and communication to large numbers of people in a matter of moments has brought great benefit but has added a different dimension to our understanding of such challenges. Leadership has, arguably, never been more important – not just from those clearly identified as 'leaders' but from 'ward to board' and by and for every one of us.

Book structure

Chapter 1. Leadership and the role of the nursing associate

In this chapter we will introduce you to some of the most relevant policies and guidelines that underpin your practice as a TNA and highlight how this can inform your understanding of the 'bigger picture'. You will be enabled to see how these impact on patient care and consider for yourself how nurses are viewed by those for whom we care. Clinical governance will be explained and placed in the context of your practice and in providing an acceptable and, hopefully, improving level of care. Finally, the leadership role of the TNA has been described including examples of key elements that underpin effective leaders.

Chapter 2. What is leadership theory and change management?

In this chapter you will be introduced to the underpinning theories and definitions of leadership and management. You will reflect on different leadership styles that you may have seen in practice and through different activities consider what type of leadership skills you possess and how you may develop your skills to lead and manage change effectively. Change management models will be presented to you along with case studies to develop your understanding of change model theory and its application to clinical practice.

Chapter 3. Understanding interpersonal skills for leadership across multiple settings

In this chapter you will explore the interpersonal skills required to provide good leadership and team-working. Good interpersonal skills may lead to satisfied, loyal and engaged teams that are able to deliver high-quality, safe and compassionate care. You will explore followership and through case studies and reflection; you may recognise the different qualities of different types of followers. The chapter will offer guidance on how you can develop your own leadership style and interpersonal skills as a TNA and on becoming an RNA.

Chapter 4. Understanding and applying the principles of human and environmental factors in relation to leadership

In this chapter you will be introduced to the concepts of human and environmental factors with definitions and examples including case studies to cite the theory in practice scenarios. No matter what environment you work in, the skills required to work effectively with your fellow human beings are similar. Activities and resources will enable you to explore these concepts and to evaluate your own non-technical skills – cognitive, social and personal – to support your situational awareness and decision-making. The chapter also helps you to appreciate that the environment in which you work is more than simply your physical surroundings and that this environment can be influenced by you as a leader.

Chapter 5. Understanding data and information for effective care and leadership

In this chapter we will explore what data and information mean for your role in healthcare. We will consider digital literacy skills, legislation, data protection and how patient data contributes to safe, effective care and evidence-informed practice. You will be given activities to consider good data management and challenge your understanding of digital safety. Additionally, we will explore how to access and share information, considering contemporary challenges in an ever-expanding digital landscape.

Chapter 6. Understanding prioritisation, workload and delegation

In this chapter we will explain the legal, ethical and professional issues that relate to prioritisation and delegation of workload. Using case studies, we will explain how the use of a matrix or triage system will ensure that work is prioritised and delegated safely. You will explore the importance of effective communication to delegate work safely as well as recognise some of the internal and external factors that may be barriers to delegation. This chapter will provide you with tools to enable you to prioritise your work effectively and delegate accordingly.

Chapter 7. Understanding how to monitor and review quality of care

In this chapter we will explore how to recognise and monitor quality of care and raise concerns when standards of care fall below expectations. We will explore the role of regulatory bodies who set examples of what good care looks like and give guidance for all health professionals to follow. To help you reflect on quality care, we will consider what negative cultures in healthcare look like and how they develop. This chapter will be supported by activities and case studies for you to access and test your critical thinking skills. Towards the end of the chapter, you should have an awareness of your role as a leader in monitoring care and the process in which it can raise concerns.

Chapter 8. Understanding compassionate leadership

As leadership is a universal skill, so is compassion a universal language – a language that all can understand and benefit from when exposed. This chapter will explain the nature of compassion, how it links to leadership and how it is a clinically impactful 'skill' that has a direct impact on patient outcomes. Relevant policies have been highlighted that underpin compassion as a requirement and not an option in healthcare and links made to professional attitudes and standards. Examples of compassionate practice have been included, such as providing focused feedback and being open and honest, and emphasis is given to the importance of self-compassion.

Requirements for the NMC: *Standards of Proficiency for Nursing Associates*

The NMC has established Standards of Proficiency to be met by applicants to different parts of the register, and these are the standards it considers necessary for safe and effective practice. This book is structured so that it will help you to understand and meet the proficiencies required for entry to the NMC register as a nursing associate. The relevant proficiencies are presented at the start of each chapter so that you can clearly see which ones the chapter addresses. The proficiencies have been designed to be generic, so apply to all fields of nursing and all care settings. This is because all nursing associates must be able to meet the needs of any person they encounter in their practice regardless of their stage of life or health challenges, whether these are mental, physical, cognitive or behavioural.

This book includes the latest Standards for 2018 onwards, taken from the *Standards of Proficiency for Nursing Associates* (NMC, 2018c).

Learning features

This series of books are specifically designed to aid learning by providing the theory and the application of theory to practice while remaining engaging. The book is separated into manageable chunks with each chapter providing theory summary boxes, specific activities, case studies, further reading and useful webpages. The book cannot provide all the information but will provide a sound background of knowledge that will enable you to develop your own learning.

You will probably find the case studies and scenarios interesting and relatable to your own practice. Reflecting on your own practices and observations will enable you to develop your leadership skills in practice.

Final word

The role of the NAs is seen as 'bridging the gap' between health and care assistants, and registered nurses. As a new role this may seem daunting to TNAs so take your time as you increase your knowledge and skills in this role. Remember to draw on the knowledge and experience of others that you work alongside as it is an essential role of all registered nurses, midwives and RNAs to support colleagues and to help them to develop their professional competence and confidence.

We hope that you find the information in this book will support your academic studies and enable you to develop your skills not only as an NA but as an effective leader.

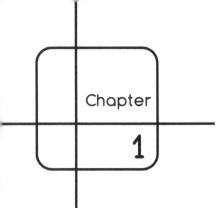

Chapter 1

Leadership and the role of the nursing associate

Sarah Tobin and
Hazel Cowls

NMC STANDARDS FOR PROFICIENCY FOR NURSING ASSOCIATES

This chapter will address the following platforms and proficiencies:

Platform 1: Being an accountable practitioner

1.1   understand and act in accordance with the Code: Professional standards of practice and behaviour for nurses, midwives and nursing associates, and fulfil all registration requirements.

Platform 4: Working in teams

4.1   demonstrate an awareness of the roles, responsibilities and scope of practice of different members of the nursing and interdisciplinary team, and their own role within it.

4.9   discuss the influence of policy and political drivers that impact health and care provision.

Platform 6: Contributing to integrated care

6.1   understand the roles of the different providers of health and care. Demonstrate the ability to work collaboratively and in partnership with professionals from different agencies in interdisciplinary teams.

Chapter aims

After reading this chapter you will be able to:

- understand the influence of policy and political drivers that impact health and care provision and why this is important;
- know what clinical governance is and how it effects patient care;
- understand the leadership role of a trainee nursing associate (TNA) and registered nursing associate (RNA).

Introduction

The National Health Service (NHS) was formed in 1948 and July 2023 will mark its 75th anniversary. Nationally the NHS is viewed positively based on the underpinning commitment to provide high-quality care available to all according to need, free at the point of delivery. There are, however, concerns about costs, staffing, an ageing population and increasing inequalities. These concerns have been heightened due to the global Covid-19 pandemic with increasing waiting times and pressures on primary and secondary care. The *NHS Long Term Plan* (2019) set out to increase funding to tackle inequalities, manage the issues experienced by staff and accelerate the redesign of patient care to future-proof the NHS for the next decade. One focus of the *NHS Long Term Plan* is the development of new roles such as that of the nursing associate (NA) as well as advanced clinical practice roles to help transform service delivery and meet the needs of the local community.

The RNA role is therefore already seen as a key addition to the healthcare workforce. The role developed because of the findings of a review, *Raising the Bar: Shape of Caring*, by Lord Willis (HEE, 2015). This review addressed the future education and training of the nursing workforce and suggested that there was a need to 'bridge' a perceived gap between the health care assistant and the registered nurse. A 2019 document from Health Education England (HEE), *Why Employ a Nursing Associate? Benefits for Health and Care Employers* (2019b), clearly states that TNAs make a great contribution to service delivery and patient care as a result of:

- improved patient communication;
- assisting nurses with a greater range of care-giving responsibilities;
- more patient-centred care and acting as a patient advocate;
- identifying and escalating patients with deteriorating health;
- displaying leadership qualities and supporting other trainees' development;
- exchanging skills, knowledge and good practice across settings, enhancing the quality of services.

As a TNA/RNA it is therefore clear that you have an important role to play in delivering care to the population and that this role encompasses the requirement to be a leader. It is possible that you may believe that you have a limited leadership role or that leadership is the preserve of those with managerial roles. The Royal College of Nurses (RCN) describes the concept of 'collective leadership' which is an assumption that leadership can and should be provided by anybody (2022a). And, while the Standards (NMC, 2018c) do not specifically describe the requirements to be a leader, they do make it clear that aspects of leadership such as supervision, delegation, providing feedback, self-management and acting as a role model are part of the role requirements. As a TNA/RNA it is important to have an understanding of the processes and structures that inform the organisations in which you work – how else can you influence how these decisions are made? And leaders should aspire to influence!

Policy and political drivers that impact health and care provision

In 2022 the Health and Care Act introduced new measures with the aim of making it simpler for all health and care providers to deliver joined-up care, especially for those people who rely on several different services. An Act of Parliament is a bill that has been approved by both the House of Commons and the House of Lords and has been given Royal Assent by the Monarch. An Act creates a new law, and this then governs what must happen in all areas that the Act covers. As an example, nurses are governed by the Health Act 1999 and a subsequent secondary legislation known as the Nursing and Midwifery Order (the Order) 2001 which forms the basis of the Nursing and Midwifery Council (NMC) Code of Conduct (2018a). It was an amendment to the 2001 Order that developed regulations which resulted in the establishment and subsequent registration of nursing associates by the NMC.

So, back to the 2022 Health and Care Act – the health needs of a population change in relation to many driving forces such as education, income, diet, employment, the environment you live in as well as the wider environment and even your own genetic makeup (known as wider determinants of health). Obviously, if healthcare provision is to stay relevant and effective this also needs to change and adapt to address these wider determinants. The Health and Care Act (2022) recognises that there are many more people living to a greater age and that these people may well have multiple health conditions that require input and ongoing support from various providers.

Activity 1.1   Research

Watch this King's Fund video (available at www.kingsfund.org.uk/audio-video/how-does-nhs-in-england-work); it lasts for 5.44 minutes.

Answer the following questions:

1. What is a 'neighbourhood' in the terms of the Health and Social Care Act 2022?
2. What is a 'place' in terms of the Health and Social Care Act 2022?
3. What are 'integrated care systems' and how many are there in England?

While you are answering these questions, consider also why this is important – what does it matter to you? The patients for whom you care will receive that care because of the decisions and even funding provided by the organisations above – it is that important and you have every right and perhaps even obligation to understand, question and influence these groups.

An outline answer is provided at the end of the chapter.

It is a common experience for many patients and of those who look after them that there is a lack of communication and integration of care between healthcare teams. Much has been written, especially in popular media, about so-called 'bed-blockers' (see Activity 1.2) and the resultant challenges of both admitting and discharging patients to and from hospitals. If one element of a system is struggling then, like so many rows of dominos, the whole system can topple. The idea to form integrated care systems stems from a wish to bring all local services that fund and support patients together – not just within the NHS but also local authorities (councils or boroughs), charities and patient groups. Cutting down on 'red tape', simplifying processes, avoiding repetition and ensuring meaningful communication across departments and organisations helps make patient care more effective and more efficient. In September 2021 the NHS set out the five principles for integrated care systems and three of the five are dedicated to supporting and developing effective leaders and leadership. The new structure designed to deliver effective healthcare makes it abundantly clear that this will only be achieved in 'an environment in which distributed leadership can thrive' (NHS England and NHS Improvement, 2021).

The Health and Care Act (2022) is a 'map' to help make it clear how care should be delivered but, in 2019, the *NHS Long Term Plan* sought to highlight how to enhance the *quality* of patient care and improve health outcomes. The plan highlighted three main priorities. First was to ensure everyone gets the best start in life by implementing measures such as reducing stillbirths and maternal deaths, increasing funding for children and young people's mental health services and improving treatments for children with cancer. The next priority was delivering 'world-class' care for major health problems including setting ambitious targets to prevent 150,000 heart attacks, strokes and cases of dementia, as well as diagnosing cancers earlier, and spending an extra £2.3 billion a year on mental health care. The third priority was to support people to age well by suggesting such initiatives as helping people to live independently at home longer, and developing more rapid community response teams to prevent unnecessary hospital admissions and speed up discharges home.

The *NHS Constitution* (Department of Health and Social Care, 2021) sets out what patients, the public and staff can expect from the NHS and what is needed from them in turn to ensure that the NHS operates fairly and effectively. There are seven principles described in the Constitution:

1. Services are comprehensive and provided to all.
2. Access to the NHS is based on need and not on an individual's ability to pay.
3. The NHS aims for the highest standards of excellence and professionalism.
4. The patient will be at the heart of everything the NHS does.
5. The NHS works across organisational boundaries.
6. The NHS will provide the best value for taxpayers' money.
7. The NHS is accountable to the public, communities and patients that it serves.

These principles are underpinned by several different values including providing respect and dignity for patients, a commitment to provide the best-quality care, improving peoples' lives by improving their health and well-being, and doing this for all to the exclusion of none and with compassion as a central element of care provision. The Constitution is, in effect, a bill of rights and sets out the obligations of the NHS to staff and patients including the responsibilities and expectations of all staff. One of these expectations is that *healthcare staff* will accept professional accountability and maintain the standards of professional practice that are set out by your professional body – in the case of an RNA this is obviously the NMC.

Activity 1.2   Reflection

The expectations and opinions of a population are influenced by experience but also by what they hear and read. Terms and headlines such as 'bed-blocker', an NHS 'in crisis', highest ever waiting lists, 'vacancies at new record level' and pictures of multiple ambulances outside hospitals are frequently presented in the UK media. This is despite legislation and policy which sets ambitious aims to improve health and social care, and dictates the formation and structure of organisations to deliver this. There is clearly a disconnect between current ambition and current provision and, at some level, this has been the case for much of the time the NHS has been in existence – it is perhaps a victim of its own success.

Having read the paragraph above – how would you seek to reassure a patient or maybe even a member of your own family who needed to seek healthcare but who was worried that their needs would not be met?

While this is a reflective exercise, some suggestions are outlined at the end of the chapter.

This section has described some very important Acts and legislation, there are many such policy documents – you cannot possibly know them all; but understanding at least some impactful regulation is helpful. You will often be working directly with patients – you and they will be resourced and governed by these policies so perhaps you ought to know what Acts dictate your acts? You are a vital component of health provision – the face of patient care – so, arguably should have a voice and an opinion that could influence the decisions made? This could be as simple as ensuring you vote in local and general elections, but there is no reason why you cannot get involved with the leadership and governance structures within your own employing organisation – what's to stop you?

What is clinical governance?

Clinical governance first emerged in the white paper *The New NHS: Modern: Dependable* (Department of Health, 1997), when it was noted that there was a degree of variation in clinical practice and outcomes across England – for example, the mortality rate for people younger than 65 years was almost three times higher in Manchester compared to West Surrey. In response to this the government introduced national standards and guidelines to produce national guidelines and audits for dissemination across healthcare organisations. At the time a new Commission for Health Improvement was established to provide support and monitor systems, processes and standards of care at a local level, later known as the Healthcare Commission. Since 2009, an independent regulatory body, the Care Quality Commission (CQC), has been responsible for maintaining standards of care in health and social care across England.

So, what is clinical governance? A widely accepted definition of clinical governance is: 'a system through which NHS organisations are accountable for continuously improving the quality of their services and safeguarding high standards of care by creating an environment in which excellence in clinical care will flourish' (Scally and Donaldson, 1998, p. 61).

More recently, Ellis (2018, p. 187) described clinical governance as: 'multiple methods of information gathering used to assess the quality of clinical care leading to improvements in the delivery and experience of care for the patient'.

All activities that promote quality, challenge and record professional practice including employees continuing professional development, any regulatory activity, audit and performance monitoring, fall within the remit of clinical governance. There are several frameworks or models that exist, although clinical governance is often thought of in terms of the *seven pillars*, which you will read about below. You will also read about the *five themes of clinical governance* (Royal College of Nursing, www.rcn.org.uk/clinical-topics/clinical-governance).

Understanding the theory: pillars of clinical governance

The *seven pillars of clinical governance* are often thought of as:

1. clinical effectiveness;
2. risk management;
3. patient and public involvement;
4. audit;
5. staff management;
6. education and training;
7. information.

The *five themes of clinical governance* (Royal College of Nursing):

1. patient focus – how the services are based on the patient needs;
2. information focus – how information is used;
3. quality improvement – how standards are reviewed and attained;
4. staff focus – how staff are developed;
5. leadership – how improvement efforts are planned.

You will note the similarities between the two examples of clinical governance, although NHS England cite the five themes as stated above (NHS England).

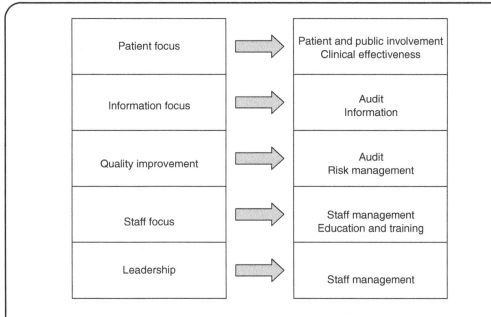

Figure 1.1 Five themes of clinical governance as applied to the seven pillars of clinical governance

For clinical governance to be effective, all stakeholders from service users and the public to clinicians, registered nurses, midwives and nursing associates, allied health professionals and trustees of health organisations need to be involved in ensuring safe practice. Registered nurses, midwives and nursing associates are well placed to ensure safe patient care and promote services that meet the needs of individuals and our communities. But how do we know we are getting it right? How do organisations and managers demonstrate that staff have the necessary skills and knowledge to perform their role? Finally, how do leaders support their staff, support their patients and provide high-quality care?

Patient focus

Patient safety is everyone's business who works in healthcare but, unfortunately, errors do occur, so it is important that individuals and organisations improve safety by reducing risk and minimising harm. At a local organisation level this may include risk assessments, safety briefings and toolbox talk. Safety briefings or toolbox talks are short talks to remind staff of any concerns or potential hazards in the workplace. Debriefings are an opportunity for staff to reflect on any tricky situations, such as patients with a challenging mental health issue or patients with complex physical ill health.

Information focus

This theme includes patient information, audit, digital literacy, data protection and legislation. In health and social care, we document care and share information as required, such as referring a person for a specific diagnostic test or specialist review.

Therefore, we need to practise the principles of General Data Protection Regulation (GDPR) by ensuring all personal data is processed lawfully and transparently, data is obtained for a specific purpose and limited only to those that need to know and handled in a way that ensures security and protection of the data (Data Protection Act, 2018).

Quality improvement

Quality improvement includes patient experience, safety and clinical effectiveness, and is a key marker of local and operational performance. There are many ways to evaluate and measure quality in health such as patient and service user feedback questionnaires, patient advice and liaison services (PALS), NHS complaints and Care Opinion. Launched in 2013, the Friends and Family Test (FFT) seeks the opinion of service users to understand what went well and where services can be improved. The same year a systematic review found a positive association between patient experience, patient safety and clinical effectiveness (Doyle et al., 2013). The review included a weight of evidence to support the patient experience, in some cases suggesting that patients can be used as partners in identifying unsafe practice and helping to develop safe, highly effective care. The CQC is an independent regulator of health and social care in England and its lines of enquiry focus on whether care is safe, effective, caring, responsive and well led (CQC, 2022). The Commissioning for Quality and Innovation (CQUIN) framework supports the improvement in the quality of services and the creation of new, improved patterns of care (NHS England, 2023). One example of a quality improvement is increasing the uptake of flu vaccinations among healthcare staff (NHS England, 2023).

In Chapter 7, you will explore how clinical audits provide a picture of how services are performing. Data collection and audit is often collated by the National Clinical Audit and Patient Outcomes Programme (NCAPOP) and the National Quality Improvement and Clinical Audit Network (NQICAN). Both networks work closely with NHS England, Healthcare Quality Improvement Partnership (HQIP) and National Institute for Health and Social Care Excellence (NICE).

Staff focus

The *NHS Constitution* (Department of Health and Social Care [DoHSC], 2021) states that the NHS will provide high-quality safe care focused on patient experience, the people it employs and the support and education that they receive. This theme refers to the safe and appropriate recruitment and management of staff in an organisation and may include the following:

1. ensuring staff have access to relevant equipment and other resources that enable them to carry out their role;
2. staff can discuss any learning needs and opportunities with their manager;
3. staff have access to relevant training;
4. staff can air any concerns with their manager or an independent person confidentially;
5. staff may need to be performance-managed.

Leadership

The *NHS Constitution* (DoHSC, 2021) states that patient safety, experience and outcomes are improved if staff feel valued, empowered and well supported. Therefore, this theme has a staff focus as well as quality assurance and performance monitoring. Quality assurance is about the maintenance of a desired level of quality in a service or product, paying attention to each stage of the process and delivery of care. Key performance indicators (KPIs) ensure that organisations can measure each process and outcome. However, KPIs will vary across all clinical areas – for example, a TNA or RNA working in primary care will have knowledge of KPIs such as health checks, health screening, immunisations and management of long-term conditions. In contrast, in urgent care the KPIs may be about time to answer a patient telephone call or time to see someone after they present to the emergency department. For clinical governance to be effective all stakeholders, from clinicians, registered nurses, midwives, health care assistants, allied health care professionals to executive boards and managers, need to understand and get involved in it. Registered nurses and midwives are key to including patients and public and promoting safety.

The following two case studies will help illustrate elements of clinical governance in practice.

Case study: Jack

Jack is a 40-year-old patient with Down Syndrome and he has a learning disability. He has been admitted to the emergency department following a fall down the stairs; he banged his head and knocked his right foot. Jack has been very reluctant to walk since. The staff in the emergency department are extremely busy and do not have time to sit with Jack. An RNA, Ali, notices that Jack looks upset and decides to sit with Jack while he waits for his parents to arrive. Ali explains the treatment plan for Jack and provides easy-read cards; he also refers Jack to the hospital learning disability team. When Jack's parents arrive, Ali takes time to explain Jack's treatment, allowing them time to ask any questions. Later, a TNA speaks to Ali, reporting that he needs to understand more about the Mental Capacity Act and asking where he can access modified assessment tools.

The *Learning Disability Improvement Standards* (NHS Improvement, 2018) have been developed by people and their families to state what they expect from the NHS. Their four standards are:

1. respecting and protecting individuals' rights;
2. inclusion and engagement for people with a learning disability, their families and carers;
3. organisations will ensure that the workforce will have specialist knowledge to support people with a learning disability, their families and carers;
4. specialist learning disability services provided by trusts.

The care delivered by Ali is in accordance with the *Learning Disability Improvement Standards* (NHS Improvement, 2018) outlined above and the scenario illustrates the following themes of clinical governance:

- *patient-focused* – as Ali takes time to sit with Jack, build a rapport and try to establish why Jack may be upset. It is important to involve the patient and their carers in any decision-making and ensure that effective communication skills are used – for example, Makaton/flash cards/easy-read cards. In this scenario, Ali has been respectful, involved Jack and his parents in his care and used appropriate language and communication to increase understanding;
- *staff-focused* – as Ali has appropriate skills to support Jack, but also within the scenario a TNA has identified that he needs to increase his knowledge.

Case study: Hilary

Hilary had been admitted to a hospital ward for investigations; recently bereaved she felt tearful and lonely. Due to the severe acute respiratory syndrome, coronavirus (SARS-CoV-2) disease or Covid-19 pandemic, the hospital restricted visiting to one person for one hour per day, but Hilary's closest relatives live approximately 250 miles away. Hilary understood that her family could not visit each day but felt isolated not having a phone to stay connected with family.

Due to restricted visiting in hospitals and care homes this was a common occurrence, with many staff reporting daily challenges by families to relax the visiting restrictions. Understandably this practice led to stress for all involved: staff, patients and their families. On this particular ward, the manager ran weekly team briefings and was supportive of staff, listening to their concerns and challenges. The team agree to provide patients with an iPad and to schedule a time when patients could contact their families. This practice was viewed positively by patients and their families.

This scenario illustrates the following themes of clinical governance:

- *patient-focused* – as there is patient and public involvement as patients now have access to iPads or other devices so that they can communicate with their families;
- *staff-focused* – by listening to staff concerns and supporting them with decisions made around visiting;
- *quality improvement* – by ensuring patients were able to communicate with family members while in hospital, therefore reducing feelings of isolation and improving the patient experience;
- *leadership* – by ensuring staff felt that they could air their concerns in a safe space.

Activity 1.3   Reflection

- What role do you play in clinical governance?
- How do you or the organisation that you work for evidence the five themes (or seven pillars) of clinical governance?

An outline answer is given at the end of this chapter.

Throughout this book we will be referring to clinical governance – for example, in Chapters 2 and 3 we will be looking at leadership theory and the interpersonal skills of a leader. Good leadership is more than managing people; it is also about how people develop their knowledge and skills. In Chapter 5 you will develop an understanding of how care-related data provides effective standards of care; in Chapter 7 you will explore how to monitor and review the quality of care delivered.

The leadership role of a trainee nursing associate and registered nursing associate

Leadership is a key skill for all nurses and care assistants and is not just restricted to those with direct managerial responsibility; this may be reiterating what we have previously said but it is very important! As an example, some staff may be leaders in their clinical role, such as an RNA leading a team or leading a wound care audit or a change in practice. The NMC (2018a, p. 21) states as a registered nurse, midwife or nursing associate 'You should be a model of integrity and leadership for others to aspire to.'

Effective leadership is essential to providing high-quality compassionate care and there has been an international drive to nurture leadership development in novice and newly qualified nurses (WHO, 2020b). All nurses need the confidence and leadership skills to be able to act as a patient advocate within the context of a multidisciplinary team (HEE, 2015). The TNA and RNA have a key role to play in leadership and followership by demonstrating effective communication skills when working in teams; providing supervision and feedback to colleagues as indicated; by improving the safety and quality of care provided (NMC, 2018a).

However, there are challenges to developing leadership skills in trainee nurses and TNAs and this is around a misunderstanding about leaders and managers as the words are often used interchangeably. As the RNA role is relatively new (NMC, 2018a), there seems to be a lack of clarity about the RNA's scope of practice and limitations to caring for patients with high levels of acuity (Lucas et al., 2021). It has been suggested that the following attributes will enable nursing students to develop their leadership skills (Jack et al., 2022) and this could also be applied to the role of the TNA:

- interpersonal competence;
- contemporary clinical knowledge;
- acting as a role model.

So, what does this look like in clinical practice? Let us look at these attributes in more detail.

Interpersonal competence

Interpersonal relates to relationships or communication with people and *competence* is having the ability to do something successfully or efficiently. Therefore, *interpersonal competence* is the ability to interact effectively with colleagues, patients, family and carers. As a TNA or RNA, practising interpersonal competence will enable you to develop a therapeutic relationship, to actively listen and provide person-centred care.

Understanding the theory: person-centred care

We have read about person-centred care and understand that person-centred care is about:

- shared decision-making;
- enabling patient choice, including their legal right to choose;
- supporting decisions made and patient self-management;
- social prescribing and community-based support;
- working in partnership with individuals and their health and social care professionals;
- personal health budgets. (NHS England, 2019)

As a leader in practice, you will be supporting and leading others such as TNAs, student nurses, healthcare or maternity support workers and need to be able to practise *interpersonal competence* in situations such as delegation or escalation of care. Effective communication with the wider professional team through delegation and supervision will lead to highly effective, safe patient care. The NMC (2018a) refers to effective communication, stating that the TNA and RNA must be able to communicate with sensitivity and compassion and be able to manage relationships that ensure safe person-centred care. The TNA and RNA need to be culturally aware of all people and ensure their preferences are considered when delivering person-centred care. These interpersonal skills will be discussed in more detail in Chapter 3 and in Chapter 8.

Contemporary clinical knowledge

As a TNA working towards registered practice, you must be able to act in the best interests of people, providing person-centred, safe and compassionate care in a range of care settings (NMC, 2018a). Contemporary clinical knowledge is about being up to date with current clinical practice: this knowledge informs us and enables us to make clinical decisions. Why is this important? The NMC (2018a) describes critical thinking and clinical decision-making as the process of analysing a situation, considering various aspects of the situation and deciding on a plan of action (or a decision). By demonstrating expertise and *contemporary clinical knowledge*, the TNA can prioritise patient care, escalate care as deemed necessary and therefore work effectively as a leader and team-worker. Throughout your foundation degree and once you qualify as an RNA you will continue to develop your knowledge; begin to recognise meaningful patterns to guide your practice; become proficient in your assessments which, in turn, improves your clinical decision-making; and be able to work as an expert within your field. This was described by Benner (2001 [1984]) as 'novice to expert'; this theory is not based on how to become a nurse but more on how a nurse develops skills and knowledge over time. See Figure 1.2.

Novice	Advanced beginner	Competent nurse	Proficient nurse	Expert
A beginner with no experience. Able to follow instructions and complete tasks	Some experience and recognises meaningful components to guide any actions	Two to three years' experience in the same role	They have a more holistic understanding of nursing, which improves decision-making	An expert nurse has experience and an intuitive grasp of clinical situations. Their performances are fluid, flexible and highly proficient

Figure 1.2   Novice to expert

Source: Adapted from Benner (2001 [1984]).

As an RNA you will continue to grow, both personally and professionally; through continuing professional development by gaining new knowledge and skills. Every three years you must revalidate with the NMC to remain on its register. Revalidation is about demonstrating good practice and provides the public with reassurance that you remain up to date in your practice (NMC, 2019b). Importantly, the process of revalidation will help you to reflect, share and improve your nursing practice.

Acting as a role model

Acting as a role model is behaving in a particular way that is observed and replicated by others. As a TNA, you are working towards registered practice and will be aware of the NMC *Code* (2018a) and the professional standards that all nurses, midwives and nursing associates must uphold to be registered to practise in the United Kingdom. *The Code* (2018a) provides a set of common standards of conduct and behaviour based around four themes; these are:

- prioritise people;
- practise effectively;
- preserve safety; and
- promote professionalism and trust.

By demonstrating these behaviours as a TNA or RNA you are acting as a role model to other nurses, midwives, nursing associates and nursing students.

Being a role model is also an important aspect of leadership in nursing, as leaders use their skills to mentor others in leading, managing their workload, effective communication skills and supporting the team and patients in their care. Examples of role modelling include demonstrating effective communication when working in teams, such as active listening when dealing with a team member's concerns or being a calm presence when exposed to a stressful situation (NMC, 2018a). This will be discussed further and in the context of compassionate leadership in Chapter 8.

Case study: Mayan

Mayan is a TNA, is on placement at a GP practice and has been working there for six weeks. Mayan is working with a health care assistant (HCA) who is running a phlebotomy clinic. The HCA has completed the appropriate venepuncture skills training and has been signed off as competent, but is feeling apprehensive about delivering their first phlebotomy clinic. Mayan is experienced and competent in venepuncture so has been asked to run the clinic with the HCA. Before starting the clinic, Mayan offers some words of encouragement and support to the HCA.

Mayan observes the HCA identify and prepare the patient for venepuncture and then carry out venepuncture as per local policy, adhering to aseptic non-touch technique (ANTT). During the procedure, the patient reported that they are prone to bleeding post venepuncture as they take antiplatelet medication, so Mayan advises the HCA to apply pressure once the needle has been removed as per local policy. Once the patient had left the clinic, Mayan gave verbal feedback to the HCA on their communication with the patient and venepuncture technique.

Activity 1.4   Reflection

The case study above illustrates that Mayan has demonstrated the three leadership skills: interpersonal skills, clinical knowledge and role modelling.

Can you recall a time when you demonstrated leadership skills such as good interpersonal skills, clinical knowledge and acting as a role model?

How can you continue to develop your skills?

As this activity is based on your own observation, there is no outline answer at the end of the chapter.

Final thought

Research on the RNA role is highlighting its importance, but there needs to be further clarity on the RNA's scope of practice. A qualitative study exploring the implementation of the RNA role in the acute setting showed some variability of the role in practice (Lucas et al., 2021). For example, some senior nurses acknowledged that the role would be beneficial to the organisation and that there was a readiness for change, whereas others cited cost implications and a lack of policy description as challenging. RNAs reported that they saw this role as an opportunity for career progression but reported challenges such as lack of understanding of the role by others and a blurring of role boundaries when staffing was poor in clinical areas.

The RNA role needs to be championed and the scope of the role clearly defined in health and social care organisations. The role should not just be seen as a career progression role, but as a role in its own right (Lucas et al., 2021). It has been recommended that TNAs and RNAs would benefit from early career development advice and support from their employers to develop their leadership skills (Robertson et al., 2022).

Chapter summary

Policy and the laws and processes that underpin healthcare delivery are extensive and, at times, complex – this chapter has introduced you to several impactful and relevant policies. An understanding of these will help you to comprehend the 'bigger picture' that establishes and constrains the care that you are able to provide. As a leader it is important to be able to influence the decision-makers and therefore to have an awareness of who the decision-makers might be. Clinical governance is a framework to ensure that standards of clinical excellence are set and then maintained, and this framework makes it very clear that effective leadership relates directly to this aim. Finally, your leadership role as a TNA/RNA has been emphasised and described, especially in relation to three elements: interpersonal skills, clinical knowledge and role modelling. This chapter introduces you to themes that will be revisited and expanded upon throughout this book.

Activities: brief outline answers

Activity 1.1 Research

The Health and Care Act 2022 created the following partnership and delivery structures:

- a 'neighbourhood' which is a network of primary care providers such as GPs, dentists, opticians and pharmacies covering a population of approximately 30,000–50,000 people;

- a 'place' which consists of health and well-being boards and place-based partnerships, which may include local authorities, Healthwatch (independent statutory body), NHS trusts and voluntary, community and social enterprise (VCSE) organisations covering a population of approximately 250,000–500,000 people;
- an 'integrated care system' made up of provider collaboratives which may be NHS trusts, the independent sector or VCSE organisations covering a population of 1–2 million people. There are 42 in England and they are made up of integrated care boards and integrated care partnerships.

Activity 1.2 Reflection

Your answer to this question will be unique and much influenced by your own engagement with healthcare, either as an employee or perhaps as a patient yourself.

It is worth noting that despite all the pressures and challenges that the NHS currently faces the Nuffield Trust reminds us that the NHS does better than other comparable countries at protecting people from excessive costs if they are ill and this, in turn, means people are not put off seeking help when needed. And, according to the American 'think tank' the Commonwealth Fund (2021), the UK ranked fourth in overall performance when compared with ten other health systems from wealthy countries in 2021. It may not be perfect, but the NHS is not failing; like any organisation, it needs funds and staff and as long as those are available in adequate numbers then evidently the NHS can and will provide adequate healthcare for the country's population.

Activity 1.3 Reflection

You may have considered the following.

1. *Patient-focused* by ensuring that patient safety is paramount, working with risk management teams and other agencies. By listening to the patient needs and designing services around this need.
2. *Information-focused* by using audit to monitor patient and staff experiences and using this to share learning from incidents and develop, maintain and monitor action plans following investigations.
3. *Quality improvement*, including the patient experience, safety and clinical effectiveness, is a key marker of operational performance in health and social care settings.
4. *Staff focus*, looking at the health and well-being of nursing staff as healthier working environments can improve patient outcomes.
5. *Leadership* styles contribute to good team-working, lower stress and higher empowerment with authentic leaders being good role models consistent with values and vision for healthcare. Leadership is a predictor of quality outcomes in healthcare settings.

Further reading

Gopee, N. and Galloway, J. (2017) *Leadership and Management in Healthcare* (3rd ed.). London: Sage.

This book covers a wide range of aspects of management and leadership particular to the healthcare environment.

West, M.A. (2021) *Compassionate Leadership: Sustaining Wisdom, Humanity and Presence in Health and Social Care*. London: Swirling Leaf Press.

An evidence-based approach to transfer leadership and cultures within health and social care teams. An insightful book that will help people think about their leadership practices.

Useful websites

www.england.nhs.uk/clinaudit/

Clinical audit: find out how NHS England uses audit to review whether healthcare is being provided in line with national standards and informs care providers and patients whether their service is doing well and where there could be improvements. Read about the National Clinical Audit and Patient Outcomes Programme (NCAPOP) and National Quality Improvement and Clinical Audit Network (NQICAN).

www.kingsfund.org.uk/health-care-explained

Health and care explained (King's Fund): videos and podcasts that explain health and care in the United Kingdom.

www.england.nhs.uk/statistics/statistical-work-areas/patient-surveys/

National patient and staff satisfaction surveys: find out how NHS England produces and uses a range of surveys to obtain feedback from patients, services users and NHS staff about the care that they receive or provide.

www.england.nhs.uk/nhs-standard-contract/cquin/cquin-23-24/

NHS England (2023) *Commissioning for Quality and Innovation (CQUIN): 2023/24*. The CQUIN framework supports improvements in the quality of services and the creation of new, improved patterns of care.

https://youtu.be/gQdV_r0poxk

An NMC-produced video on what revalidation means for nurses, midwives and nursing associates.

https://www.england.nhs.uk/sustainableimprovement/qsir-programme/qsir-tools/

Quality, service improvement and redesign (QSIR) tools – a collection of service improvement and redesign tools that can be applied to a wide variety of situations.

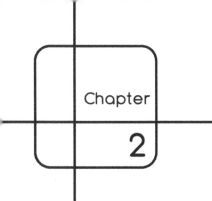

Chapter 2

What is leadership theory and change management?

Hazel Cowls

NMC STANDARDS FOR PROFICIENCY FOR NURSING ASSOCIATES

This chapter will address the following platforms and proficiencies

Platform 1: Being an accountable practitioner

1.1   understand and act in accordance with the Code: Professional standards of practice and behaviour for nurses, midwives and nursing associates, and fulfil all registration requirements.

Platform 4: Working in teams

4.1   demonstrate an awareness of the roles, responsibilities and scope of practice of different members of the nursing and interdisciplinary team, and their own role within it.

4.2   demonstrate an ability to support and motivate other members of the care team and interact confidently with them.

4.7   support, supervise and act as a role model to nursing associate students, health care support workers and those new to care roles, review the quality of the care they provide, promoting reflection and providing constructive feedback.

Annexe A: Communication and relationship management skills

4.   Demonstrate effective communication skills for working in professional teams.

Chapter aims

After reading this chapter you will be able to:

- understand the difference between leadership and management;
- explore leadership and management theory and followership in the healthcare setting;
- explore change management models and their application to practice.

Introduction

In Chapter 1 you looked at which policy and political drivers affect health and social care provision. It is recognised that the National Health Service (NHS) is built on a set of principles that bind together individuals, the people it serves and the people it employs (DoHSC, 2021).

In order to provide evidence-based, high-quality patient care, the NHS alone employs 1,257,395 full-time equivalent positions across NHS hospitals and community health services across England (NHS Digital, 2022) and is viewed as one of the world's largest employers of skilled professionals (NHS England, 2019). The NHS has pledged to provide a positive working environment, to support all staff and ensure that they have access to further education or training to enable them to achieve their full potential (DoHSC, 2021). Furthermore, with health and social care provision constantly adapting to the needs of individuals and communities, staff are encouraged to consider alternative ways of working that may improve patient services (DoHSC, 2021).

Contemporary leadership in healthcare is viewed as something that could be undertaken by the most appropriate person, regardless of their levels of responsibility or profession (Gordon et al., 2015), as this has been shown to improve patient outcomes, improve safety and improve staff morale (King's Fund, 2012). However, reports of failings in leadership in healthcare resulting in patient suffering and harm have raised questions about the apparent theory/practice gap (Francis, 2013). It is therefore important for all people working in health to understand the underpinning principles of leadership and change management theory, to be able to support leaders and followers and work collaboratively.

In this chapter, you will explore leadership and management theories in the healthcare setting. You will reflect on different leadership styles that you may have seen in practice. You will consider what type of leadership skills you possess and how you may develop your own skills to lead and manage change effectively. You will explore change model theory and its application to clinical practice.

Brief history of leaders

Leadership is not a 20th- or 21st-century concept; throughout history we have read about different leaders, from Confucius (551–479 BCE), a Chinese philosopher and politician, and Alexander the Great (356–323 BCE), a military leader from Macedonia, to Mahatma Ghandi (1869–1948), an Indian civil rights leader, and Winston Churchill (1874–1965), an army officer and Prime Minister of the United Kingdom. All these leaders, as well as countless others like them, will be remembered for their leadership and decision-making.

So, what makes a person a leader? Are leaders born or are they created? A leader needs a vision or a goal, something that is going to meet with agreement from others. A leader will possess qualities such as confidence and charisma. They will be a negotiator, a delegator, a person who is willing to take risks. The leader will also need followers with whom they can share the vision and to whom they delegate tasks to implement the vision. We will review followership later in this chapter (and Chapter 3), but first let us consider the definitions of leadership and management.

Defining leadership and management

Are there differences between a leader and a manager? Often these words are used synonymously and both words have been debated in many journals, books and webpages, each providing a variety of definitions of leadership and management. The definitions of leadership may describe the fundamental qualities of a leader and the leaders' relationships within teams or groups of people – for example, a leader is 'a person who leads a group of people, especially the head of a country, an organization, etc.' (*Oxford Learner's Dictionary*, n.d.). Whereas Northouse (2019, p. 2) stated that as soon as 'we try to define leadership, we immediately discover that leadership has many different meanings'. Buchanan and Huczynski (2019) later defined leadership as the process of *influencing* activities undertaken by the team such as goal setting and goal achievement.

The terms 'manager' and 'management' refer to the actions of a person or persons who will take control of situations and maintain the status quo which involves exercising formal authority in the workplace (Atsalos and Greenwood, 2001; Callaghan, 2007). One definition of a manager is 'a person who is in charge of running a business, a shop or a similar organization or part of one' (*Oxford Learner's Dictionary*, n.d.), suggesting that a manager is focused on the needs and goals of the organisation. Drucker (2007, p. 6) defined a manager as 'someone who directs the work of others and who does his work by getting other people to do theirs', suggesting that the manager is responsible for the work that is carried out by the employees. In nursing circles, the role of manager has been given more attention than that of a leader (Atsalos and Greenwood, 2001), with many nurses and nursing theorists using the words interchangeably and, by doing so, suggesting that it may only be the manager that can lead (Grossman and Valiga, 2012).

Leaders and managers

In practice, leadership and management may look quite different as a unit or departmental manager may have designated authority and the role will form part of the organisational hierarchy. The manager will be responsible for planning and organising both people (human resources) and resources such as medical consumables, pharmaceuticals and other medical goods. In contrast, a leader may not have designated authority or formal budgeting responsibilities, but a leader will develop interpersonal relationships and empower team members (Marquis and Huston, 2012).

Look at Table 2.1; do you notice similarities and notable differences in leadership and management skills?

Table 2.1   Skills for leadership and management

Leadership	Management
Planning	Planning
Organising	Organising
Role modelling	Staffing
Effective communication	Effective communication
Motivating others	Controlling
Delegating	Business skills
Being knowledgeable	Leading
Maintaining team dynamics	Professionalism
Supporting	Workforce planning
Decision-making	Recruiting
Visionary	Performance management and appraisal
Professionalism	Employer well-being
Coaching	Directive

Some of the skills from Table 2.1 focus on how an organisation is run, such as planning, organising, workforce planning, recruitment, appraisals and directives, while other skills focus on personnel development, interpersonal skills and change management. There are also overlapping skills for leaders and managers as both need to be professional, organised, able to lead and possess excellent communication skills. So, are leaders and managers able to co-exist?

In healthcare leaders are traditionally viewed as holding a management position such as a ward manager, deputy ward manager or outpatient manager, but this is not the case as leaders do not need to hold a formal leadership role. Many registered nurses (RN), midwives (MW) and RNAs act in a leadership position every day but may not always recognise these activities as leadership roles or that they are demonstrating leadership skills. For example, an RN 'in charge' of a ward is acting in a leadership role and will ensure that staff are delivering safe care.

Case study: Fredik

Fredik, a second-year TNA, and Timothy, a first-year TNA, are working on a community assessment ward for patients with mental health illness. A young woman has been admitted to the ward as she is to commence new medication and needs to be observed for the first dose. Fredik is completing a patient assessment document and Timothy is observing. The young woman has lots of questions about the proposed treatment. Fredik does not have all the answers so explains this and informs her that he will let the admitting doctor know and he will be able to answer all her questions.

Activity 2.1   Reflection

- What leadership qualities can you identify in this case study?
- Can you also list other leadership qualities seen in nursing, midwifery, RNA and trainee nursing/TNA roles?
- Can you recall a time in practice when you have acted as a leader? What did you do and how did that make you feel?

Some of this activity is based on your own observation, but an outline answer is given at the end of this chapter.

What are leadership theories and leadership styles?

Understanding leadership theory and leadership styles will enable individuals to recognise their own qualities and develop their skills in leadership and in Chapter 3 you will consider your own leadership style. Leadership theories and leadership styles are often intertwined (Figure 2.1). However, leadership theory focuses on the characteristics, qualities and behaviours of individuals, as well as the circumstances that will enable them to be successful leaders, whereas leadership styles describe the actions that leaders adopt to achieve short- and long-term goals, such as coaching, working collaboratively and with vision. Leadership styles sit under the umbrella of leadership theory. In this section, we will discuss the differences between leadership theory and leadership styles.

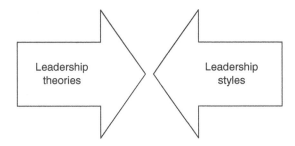

Figure 2.1   Leadership theories and styles

Each theory describes the specific qualities of the leader and how they interact with others. An outline of each theory is briefly explained in the 'Understanding the theory' box below. You may recognise patterns, skills and behaviours of leaders in practice across the health and social care setting.

Understanding the theory: leadership theories

Great Man Theory

First mentioned in 1897 by Carlyle, who suggested that leaders are born, not made – for example, royalty or people working in the Church or politics.

Trait Theory

Like *great man* this suggests that individuals will show specific qualities or characteristics suiting them to leadership roles such as ambition, assertiveness, confidence or decisiveness (Stogdill, 1974). Initial research into the traits of leaders and non-leaders highlighted minor variances between the two (Burns and West, 2003).

Contingency Theory

Also termed *situational* theory. Contingency leadership theory suggests that leaders do not change: it is the environment and team dynamics that change. Contingency theory and situational theory focus on the relationship between the leader, the subordinates and the environment or situation (Bass, 1992). For example, an authoritarian style may be appropriate when the leader is the most knowledgeable and experienced, whereas a democratic approach to leadership may prove effective in groups consisting of skilled experts. The leader will adapt and make decisions based on the current situation, the team and the organisation. An example to illustrate this is a leader who had to facilitate change and support the team during the Covid-19 pandemic.

Behaviour Theory

In behaviour leadership theory, the personal traits of a leader provide the foundation for leadership with leaders drawing on prior experience. This leader has developed leadership knowledge and skills over time and recognises that one style of leadership may not be suited to all situations. This leader will actively seek the opinion of others to continually develop their own leadership skills. For example, requesting anonymous 360° feedback from superiors and colleagues. Weber (1905) described two types of leaders as *bureaucratic* and *charismatic*; the bureaucratic leader will follow policies and procedures, so is well suited to large organisations such as the National Health Service. In contrast, a charismatic leader will lead through enthusiasm and motivation.

Participative Theory

Also termed *democratic* leadership theory. Focuses on the input and contribution of others. In the 1930s studies were conducted by Kurt Lewin, who identified this type of leadership in organisations (Bass and Avolio, 1995). Individuals are involved in decision-making processes, although the leader retains the right to control member input. This leader will arrange a team meeting and encourage colleagues to share ideas. As a result, staff feel well informed; this type of leadership will improve staff morale and encourage collaborative working.

Management Theory

Also termed *transactional*, this theory assumes that a person does not have to be a natural leader to be in this position. A transactional leader is leading by virtue due to the management position that they hold in an organisation. Transactional leaders aim to maintain an equilibrium and harmony by ensuring that the organisational goals are met according to the policies and procedures and that teams are rewarded on performance (Bass and Riggio, 2006). The leader will focus on coaching followers and ensuring that they have the appropriate skills and access to training to fulfil the organisational objectives.

Relationship Theory

Also termed *transformational*, this theory was first described by James MacGregor Burns. Burns (1978) suggested that leadership is about the connections formed between leaders and their followers. The transformational leader will motivate and inspire followers and teams to develop their ideas, enabling them to fulfil their potential as well as group performance. The leader merges their own goals and followers' goals with the overall organisational objectives. Burns' thoughts were extended by Bernard M. Bass, who described four components in transformational leadership: ideal impact, intellectual stimulation, personal consideration and strong motivation (Tucker and Russell, 2004). This type of leader is thought to have high ethical and moral standards (Burns and West, 2003) and is recognised as a leader who will actively listen to the views of the whole team before any decisions are finalised.

Two of the most successful leadership theories are transactional leadership (management theory) and transformational leadership (relationship theory). A transactional approach to leadership in healthcare can be advantageous as this type of leadership aims to maintain the status quo by following organisational policies and procedures; however, there is also a need for a transformational leadership as a transformational leader will engage with the team, inspire followers and empower followers to achieve their best. To deliver a complex, safe, evidence-based health service the leaders need to implement local and national policy, but also strive for excellence and make changes where necessary to maintain safe care and receive positive patient feedback. Therefore, a combination of transactional and transformational leadership would be appropriate. Table 2.2 illustrates the differences between both leadership approaches.

Activity 2.2   Research

Read around the topic of leadership and management in health and social care. From the list above choose four leadership theories and consider the strengths and weaknesses of each leadership theory.

The aim of this activity is to develop a deeper understanding of leadership theory, to recognise the strengths and limitations of at least four leadership theories. There is no outline answer at the end of this chapter.

Table 2.2   Difference between transactional and transformational leaders

Transactional leadership theory	Transformational leadership theory
Leader focuses on organisational goals	Awareness of organisational goals, but will look at merging own goal and others
Leader is task-centred and will follow organisational and national policies and procedures	
Short- and medium-term goals	Inspires followers to believe in themselves and to develop their ideas
Focus on self and organisation	Will empower followers to be creative
A coach but expects people to follow the lead	Interested in the organisation but also welcomes innovation
	Encourages individual growth
Reward system	Rewards informally

Leadership in the NHS requires leaders to lead with care and compassion. In 2013, the NHS Leadership Academy developed the Healthcare Leadership model (Storey and Holti, 2013). There are three key elements that underpin the NHS Leadership Model: first, to provide and justify a clear sense of purpose and contribution that focuses on the needs of the service users; second, to motivate teams by building on team commitment, encouraging staff engagement, managing and improving staff performance as well as listening to staff; and, finally, focusing on systems and service improvement, initiating new structures and processes and new ways of working (Storey and Holti, 2013). These elements link clearly to the values of the NHS by ensuring individuals and teams provide a comprehensive service to all and that the patient is at the heart of everything that it does (DoHSC, 2021). You will have explored the policies and political drivers that have influenced health and social care in Chapter 1, recognising that papers such as *Liberating the NHS* (DoHSC, 2010), the Francis Report (Francis, 2013) and *Raising the Bar: The Shape of Caring* (HEE, 2015) have been instrumental in health service reforms and emphasising the role of the leader in providing safe patient care.

The foundations of the Healthcare Leadership model (NHS Leadership Academy, 2013) sit with relationship theory as this model focuses on the individual, their interpersonal skills and about the people they are working alongside. There are nine dimensions to this model: leading with care, sharing the vision, influencing for results, engaging the team, evaluating information, inspiring shared purpose, connecting our service, developing capability and holding to account (Storey and Holti, 2013). In Chapter 3 you will research the Healthcare Leadership model.

What are leadership styles?

As mentioned above, leadership theories and leadership styles are terms that are used synonymously but there are subtle differences; a leadership style refers specifically to the characteristics displayed by a leader when coaching, directing, guiding and managing groups of people. Individuals working across health and social care will apply distinctive styles of leadership or management at various times, depending on the situation, the goal and the team. In the late 1930s, psychologist Kurt Lewin first described three primary leadership/management styles that have provided the foundation for leadership styles from that day forward. These were authoritarian (autocratic), participative (democratic) and delegative (laissez-faire) leader.

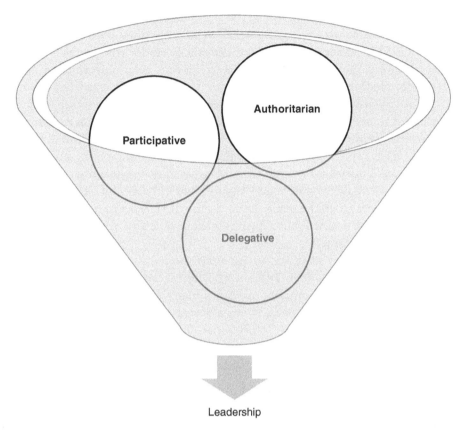

Figure 2.2   Leadership styles

Source: Adapted from Lewin et al. (1939).

Understanding the theory: leadership styles

- An authoritarian or autocratic leader exercises a position of power and authority. The leader will control and direct others, often making decisions alone. An authoritarian leader expects obedience from others.
- A participative or democratic leader will actively seek the opinion and involvement of the team. A participative leader will work with individuals and the teams and encourages collaborative teamwork.
- A delegative or laissez-faire leader appears relaxed about rules and policies. The delegative leader allows members freedom of choice and intervenes only when approached or when a crisis is evident. A delegative leader monitors performance from a distance and can appear detached from the team and individuals.

Other leadership styles include an *affiliative* leader, a *bureaucratic* leader, a *coercive* leader, a *commanding* leader, a *pacesetting* leader and a *visionary* leader. The characteristics shown by leaders will influence individuals, the team as well as the organisation's culture. For example, an *affiliative* leader will motivate others even during challenging times and create harmony in the workplace. A *bureaucratic* leader is viewed as impersonal, someone who follows established policies and rules and expects the staff to do the same. This leader is viewed as inflexible. A leader who *coaches* will nurture the team by helping employees look at ways to improve their performance. A *coercive* leader provides clear direction in crisis situations but requires immediate compliance all the time. A *commanding* leader who is forceful will often make tough or unpopular decisions but at times this may be what is needed for an organisation such as during a pandemic when it is important for a leader to take control of the situation. A *pacesetting* leader will set high standards and expects the team to be highly motivated and always deliver excellence. This leader is most effective when quick results are required. Finally, a *visionary* leader who is innovative and imaginative will drive forward change and will encourage their peers to do the same. In doing this it is likely to be a positive place to work and the organisation will have high retention of staff – plus, happy staff equals happy patients (Gopee, 2022).

Another way of looking at this is to consider the language used by leaders when they are managing change (see Table 2.3). The leadership styles that promote a positive organisational environment are more likely to create change; arguably the pacesetters and commanding leaders can also facilitate change, but there may be more resistance to the change. We will look at change management theory later in this chapter.

Table 2.3   Leadership styles and the climate they support

Leadership styles that may lead to a positive organisational environment	Leadership styles that may lead to a negative organisational environment
Visionary leaders say *'come with me'*	Pacesetting leaders set high standards and say to their followers *'do what I do now'*
Coaching facilitates performance and leaders say *'try this'*	
Affiliative leaders build emotional connections and say *'people come first'*	Commanding leaders are authoritative, with leaders saying *'do what I tell you'*
Democratic leaders work on building consensus and shared decision-making by saying *'what do think?'*	

Source: Adapted from Goleman (2000).

Activity 2.3   Critical thinking

You have reviewed different leadership styles and have seen different leaders in your clinical practice. Either in a group or individually, please draw up a list of pros and cons on each of the following leadership styles:

1. autocratic;
2. democratic;
3. laissez-faire.

An outline answer is given at the end of this chapter.

Activity 2.4 Reflection

Take a moment to reflect on a leader or manager that you admire. Do you think you could inspire others as much as they have inspired you? How would you inspire others? What obstacles do you see that would keep you from being a great leader?

As this activity is based on your own observation, there is no outline answer at the end of the chapter.

Followership

We cannot write about leadership and management theories without mentioning *followership* as the three are intrinsically linked, each depending on the others (see Figure 2.3, which illustrates the leadership triad). Traditionally, followers have been as a recipient of a leader or manager, someone who will carry instructions on behalf of the leader/manager, often seen as subservient to a manager or leader – although Shamir (2007) suggested that followership is as important as leading or managing and negates the idea of shared leadership.

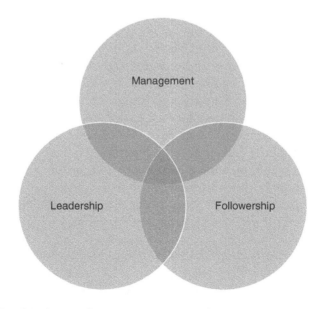

Figure 2.3 A leadership and management triad

According to Uhl-Bien et al. (2014, p. 83), 'leadership can only occur if there is followership - without followers and following behaviors there is no leadership'. The majority of the NHS workforce is made of followers – approximately 80 per cent (Crawford and Daniels, 2014) – so, unsurprisingly, followership has been studied in more detail. A review of literature identified the importance of the relationship between leaders and followers and that most people working in health will have worked or continue to work in a followership role (Leung et al., 2018). Furthermore, the review recognised different followership styles (discussed in Chapter 3) and that these styles will affect individuals' as well as organisational performance. Specifically, a follower with a higher level of critical thinking and engagement is more likely to achieve job satisfaction and personal goals (Leung et al., 2018).

An introduction to managing change

Change in health and social care is essential to improve and develop services to the needs of individuals and communities. There can be many reasons for implementing change such as new medication, treatments, care pathways, a patient complaint. Change can be delivered in different ways:

- imposed by the manager;
- managed by a designated person;
- introduced gradually following team meetings;
- evolve over time.

But who is more effective in leading and managing change in an organisation? You could argue that it depends on the situation, the change being brought about and the key stakeholders. Table 2.4 illustrates how leaders and managers differ when it comes to managing change. We will look at change management models later in this chapter.

In Table 2.4, you will note that the leader and a manager will adopt a different approach. The factors that may influence their approach depend upon their role, their leadership style, the change being implemented and the urgency of the change. Since 2020, we have seen several changes in clinical practice prompted by the Covid-19 pandemic forcing health and social care organisations throughout the world to introduce changes that would reduce the transference of the virus (WHO, 2020a). Among the biggest changes seen were visiting restrictions at hospitals, nursing homes, residential homes and surgeries. These needed to be implemented quickly to reduce the transfer of the pathogen so it would be appropriate for a manager (or transactional leader) to lead the change, bringing order and consistency to the change.

But visiting restrictions were not the only changes we saw in health and social care. Some other examples that you may have seen are as follows:

- use of personal protective equipment such as gloves, face masks, aprons, visors;
- changes to cardio-pulmonary resuscitation (CPR) techniques;
- increase in online or telephone consultations with GP or clinical specialists;
- use of digital technology to reduce patient isolation in nursing homes.

Table 2.4 Leadership and management in the context of change and movement

	Leadership produces change and movement	Management produces order and consistency
Organisation	Establishing direction	Planning and budgeting
	Creating a vision	Establishing agendas
	Selling strategies	Setting timetables
		Allocating resources
People	Aligning people	Organising staff
	Communicating goals	Providing structure
	Seeking commitment	Establishing rules and procedures
	Building teams and coalitions	
Moving the change forward	Motivating and inspiring	Controlling and problem-solving
	Empowering	Developing incentives
	Energising	Generating creative solutions
	Satisfying unmet needs	Taking corrective action

Source: Adapted from Kotter (1990).

Many of these changes happened overnight and with little time for planning; this brought about new challenges. Some of the challenges could have been due to:

- lack of time to communicate and share the vision;
- lack of time to plan the change;
- no regular review of the change;
- possible varying practices nationwide.

The following challenges were highlighted when moving face-to-face consultations with GPs to remote consultations, either telephone or video consultations:

- adapting to a new way of working for the service user and clinician;
- exposure of the limitations of IT infrastructure within the NHS as service users reported it as ineffective (55 per cent);
- ineffective IT software (52 per cent);
- use of mobile devices/apps (52 per cent);
- reduced internet speed or bandwidth (50 per cent) (BMA, 2022).

It is likely that most of these large-scale changes required a transactional and transformational approach to ensure changes were made but also that staff were supported throughout the change process. In contrast, to the large-scale changes, a relatively small project introducing the use of smart bluetooth speakers (e.g., Echo Dot) in nursing homes to improve residents' well-being would require a transformational leader to create a vision, communicate the idea, seek commitment from the team and continue to motivate people to move the change forward (Edwards et al., 2021).

Inevitably, whenever there is change people involved may feel excited by the change, or apprehensive, or threatened. It is especially important that there is a leader to manage the change process. There are a few published models of change such as Lewin's three-stage process (1951), Kotter's eight-stage model (1995), Plan–Do–Study–Act (PDSA) model (IHI, 2016) and RAPSIES (Gopee and Galloway, 2017) that will be discussed later in this chapter.

Change model theory

The management of change in any environment is not without challenges but a change model provides a framework that enables effective change to occur (Shaw, 2007). The role of the leader of change (known as a change agent) is to identify, first, if change is required. There are three questions that need to be asked:

1. what are we trying to accomplish?
2. how will we know the change is an improvement?
3. what changes can we make that will result in an improvement?

Lewin (1951) wrote extensively about change theory and suggested that the behaviour in any organisation is not static but a constant movement of socio-psychological forces working in opposite directions. A force field analysis (FFA) exercise that identifies factors that may drive or hinder change can be undertaken by an individual or a team and can be useful to 'unfreeze' the current status quo (stage one of Lewin's three-stage process of change model). To illustrate Lewin's FFA, let us look again at the SARS-CoV-2 virus (Covid-19) pandemic and the proposed change to restrict visiting to hospitals, care homes and general practice to reduce the transference of the virus. Table 2.5 highlights the driving and potential restraining forces to implementing visiting restrictions.

Table 2.5 Force field analysis

Driving force	The proposed change	Restraining force
Reduce transference of SARS-CoV-2 pathogen	Restricted visiting in hospitals, care homes and general practice	Staff not wanting to change
Reduce numbers of patients contracting SARS-CoV-2 disease requiring hospitalisation		Patients and residents want to see their family
Reduce numbers of patients admitted to hospital that may/may not require critical care bed		Risk of increasing social isolation
Reduce numbers of healthcare staff contracting SARS-CoV-2		Risk of increasing mental health concerns for individuals due to social isolation
Maintain a workforce to care in healthcare settings		
Maintain a workforce to care for people with SARS-CoV-2 and other health problems		

Source: Adapted from Lewin (1951).

The FFA for restricted visiting illustrates several drivers and restrictors for change, but it is clear from this diagram that the driver for change, such as reducing the transference of the disease, reducing ill-health, reducing mortality, protecting NHS beds outweighs the restrictors for change.

Lewin's three-stage process of change (Lewin, 1951)

Lewin's three-stage model was introduced in the early 1950s. The first stage of Lewin's three-stage model of change is to create the right environment for change by recognising the need for change and by providing a clear rationale, including evidence to support the proposed change (see FFA above). The second stage is to support the change to a desired state by involving key stakeholders, such as service providers and service users, throughout the change process. This is achieved by liaising with stakeholders, seeking opinions and sharing progress. The final stage is to reinforce or anchor the change so that it is maintained in practice. This is achieved by constant review of the change and feedback from stakeholders.

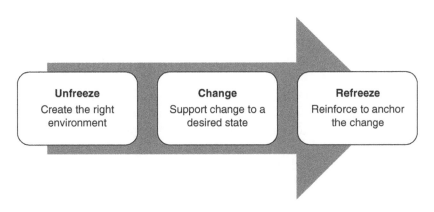

Figure 2.4   Unfreeze/change/refreeze model

Source: Adapted from Lewin's three-stage process (1951).

Kotter's eight-stage model (Kotter, 1995)

Kotter suggested that approximately 70 per cent of large-scale change is not successful because of barriers to change such as lack of engagement from the team, a lack of communication about the change to relevant people, no plan to implement the change and organisational culture. Kotter described an eight-stage model (see Figure 2.5).

The first stage is to create a sense of urgency by examining what needs to change – the opportunities as well as the challenges. Stage two is about building a coalition, or a group of people, that can lead the change. The third stage is forming a strategic vision to ensure that this becomes a reality. The fourth stage is to communicate the vision and enlist help from key people. The fifth stage is to enable action by eliminating any obstacles and changing existing processes and structures that may inhibit the proposed change.

The sixth stage is to generate short-term wins to showcase improvements and to encourage motivation. Stage seven refers to the consolidation of change and encouraging people to embrace the change and support the process. The final stage is anchoring the new change and embedding it into current practices (McKinney and Morris, 2010).

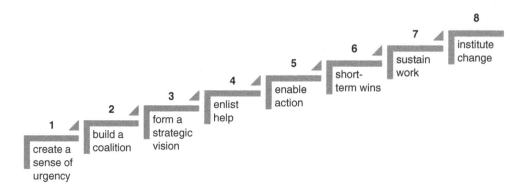

Figure 2.5   Kotter's 8–stage model

Source: Adapted from Kotter (1995).

Plan-Do-Study-Act (PDSA) model (IHI, 2016)

The Plan–Do–Study–Act (PDSA) model (IHI, 2016), also known as Demming cycle, is a quality improvement model consisting of four steps and often used in healthcare (Taylor et al., 2013). The steps to implementing change are sequential and may be repeated while the change is being implemented. The cycle appears to be simple, promotes continuing improvements and involves others, therefore reducing potential barriers to change (Gopee and Galloway, 2017). However, a systematic review of the cycle found that there was a lack of adherence to following the steps and limited progression of cycles (Taylor et al., 2013).

Seven-step RAPSIES model (Gopee and Galloway, 2017)

RAPSIES model is a seven-step approach developed by Gopee and Galloway (2017). The first step is to recognise the need for change such as to solve a problem or improve an element of practice. The second step is to analyse the options available that will improve the change, the environment or setting where the change may be implemented. The third step is to prepare for the change by identifying an appropriate person (a change agent) who may lead the implementation of change by liaising with key stakeholders and providing education to the users of the change. The fourth step is developing strategies to implement the change, leading to the fifth step, which is the implementation of the change, including piloting the change and reviewing the timing of implementation. The sixth step is to evaluate the impact of the change against the agreed and intended outcomes. The final step is to sustain the change, ensuring that the change is embedded into current practice.

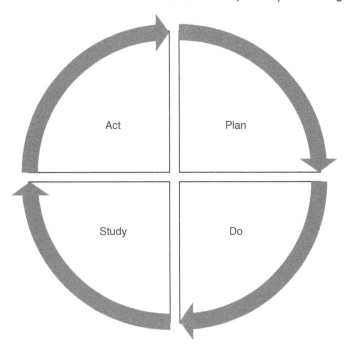

Figure 2.6 PDSA model

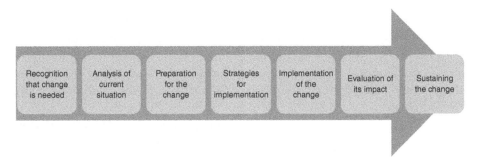

Figure 2.7 Seven-step RAPSIES model

Source: Gopee (2010, version from Gopee, 2022).

Understanding the theory: comparing the models of change

Each model of change has a series of steps but there are similarities between the models, see below.

(Continued)

(Continued)

Table 2.6 A comparison of three models of change

Lewin three-stage model (1951)	Kotter's eight-stage model (1995)	Seven-step RAPSIES model (2017)
Unfreeze	Create a sense of urgency	Recognition
	Build a coalition	Analysis
	Form a strategic vision	Preparation
	Enlist help	Strategies
Change	Enable action	Implementation
	Short-term wins	Evaluation
	Sustain work	
Freeze	Institute change	Sustaining

Understanding the theory: applying the theory to practice scenario

It has been shown that community teams tend to employ smaller numbers of TNAs compared to hospital trusts (Kessler et al., 2021). The Children and Adolescent Mental Health Services (CAMHS) Learning Disability team are looking to recruit RNAs to their team as the senior nurses recognise the benefits of employing an RNA. The RNA will take part in the assessment of young people with a learning disability and complex mental health needs. The RNA will be expected to work with the young person, families or carer in an environment suitable for the young person. The RNA will attend case reviews and work alongside other healthcare professionals working within the CAMHS Learning Disability team.

As this is a new deployment, the change will be brought about using the PDSA change model. The first step is to ask the following questions:

1. what are we trying to accomplish?
2. how will we know the change is an improvement?
3. what changes can we make that will result in an improvement?

Using the PDSA model, the following steps are completed:

- *Plan*: The manager will meet with the business manager and write a business case for the new role. The manager will clearly explain the role of the RNA to the team and other stakeholders. The manager will secure funding to advertise and appoint a TNA and RNA to the CAMHS Learning Disability team.
- *Do*: Deployment of the RNA; the RNA will be allocated a mentor. The RNA will attend regular progress reviews.

- *Study*: Obtain feedback from the RNA, wider team and other stakeholders. Review all data.
- *Act*: Connect to the patient journey; is this making a difference and how? Depending on the data collected, may need to go back to the plan, do, study and act.

This is a simple illustration of how a change can be brought about using a change model.

Activity 2.5   In Practice

1. You are an RNA working on an acute mental health unit. You are interested in sustainable healthcare and wish to set up a 'green walking group'. Although walking groups are an established intervention in acute mental healthcare, they are rarely utilised. Providing a space for patients to spend time in green spaces can promote general well-being and improve physical health.

Using a change model, what steps could you take to implement this change in practice?

2. Reflect on a recent change that you may have seen in your workplace.

What was the change? Who was involved? How was this change in practice managed?

Do you recognise a specific change model that was used to implement the change?

Could this change in practice have been managed better and, if so, how?

An outline answer is given at the end of this chapter.

Chapter summary

This chapter has explored the similarities and differences between leadership and management. A manager will be focused on the needs and goals of an organisation, and will be responsible for budgeting, planning and ensuring staff have the necessary skills. In contrast, a leader may not have designated authority within the organisation but will be developing relationships and empowering others to develop. The literature suggests that there are different leadership theories and styles, often overlapping. Remember, the leader does not need to be a person with designated authority to make a change in practice. Change management models have been discussed since the early 1950s and are constantly evolving. Change management models are a structured approach that can help the leader plan and implement a change in practice. The literature suggests that there are different change management models that focus on the process of change as well as the people who can facilitate the change.

Activities: brief outline answers

Activity 2.1

The leadership skills identified in this case study are:

- carrying out patient assessments, implementing and planning high-quality, safe patient care;
- communicating effectively with the patient and their family;
- acting as a role model to the immediate nursing team.

Other examples of nursing leadership are as follows:

- acting as a role model for the wider multidisciplinary team (MDT);
- liaising with the wider MDT;
- planning and coordinating meetings (e.g., team meeting; MDT meeting, training/skills meeting);
- being able to lead a clinical audit and encouraging others to complete the audits;
- leading a team to achieve a goal;
- leading a local project.

Activity 2.3

You may have produced the following pros and cons list for each leadership style:

Leadership	Pros	Cons
Autocratic	Directive, effective in an emergency setting, hierarchical relationship	Inflexible, authoritarian, controlling
Democratic	Inclusive, trusting relationship, encourages creativity, problem-solving	Procrastination, uncertainty, leaders can feel overwhelmed
Laissez-faire	Leaders encourage growth, innovation, increased job satisfaction	Laziness, low productivity, complacency, reduced accountability

Activity 2.5

As discussed in this chapter there are several different change models; here we have provided an answer using two different models.

1. Lewin's unfreeze/change/refreeze model

Steps	Action
Step 1 Create a sense of urgency	The leader creates the right environment for change. The change is supported with evidence on 'green walking' and shared with the team. Meet with colleagues to discuss how change can be brought about.

Steps	Action
Step 2 Support the change to a desired state	The leader would check in with service users and healthcare professionals, obtain feedback and feedforward. The leader could delegate some tasks to other people within the team.
Step 3 Reinforce to anchor the change	The leader would promote change and continually review the change.

2.   Kotter's eight-stage model

This change model focuses on people and how a team of people can help drive a change forward using the eight stages of Kotter's model. This model is methodical; all stages of this model need to be completed to increase the likelihood of a successful change.

Stages	Action
Create a sense of urgency	Provide the team with a rationale for change, support with evidence on 'green walking'.
Build a coalition	Meet with the team to discuss the proposed change.
Form a strategic vision	Continue to build on the coalition by agreeing a strategic plan with a group of people (e.g., set goals for implementation of 'green walking').
Enlist help	Enlist help and delegate specific tasks to individuals to help drive the change forward (e.g., risk assessment).
Enable action	Provide the team with resources or time to enable action.
Short-term wins	Celebrate short-term wins with the team and key stakeholders as this maintains momentum (e.g., arrange a short 'green walk', obtain and share any feedback).
Sustain the work	Keep going with the strategic plan, obtain feedback and feedforward from stakeholders.
Institute the change	Finally, the change becomes embedded in clinical practice.

Further reading

Benmira, S. and Agboola, M. (2021) Evolution of leadership theory. *BMJ Leader*, 5(1). https://bmjleader.bmj.com/content/5/1/3

This free journal article explores the historical evolution of significant leadership theories.

Harrison, R., Fischer, S., Walpola, R.L., Chauhan, A., Babalola, T., Mears, S. and Le-Do, H. (2021) Where do models for change management, improvement and implementation meet? A systematic review of the applications of change management models in healthcare. *Journal of Healthcare Leadership*, 13: 85–108.

A review of the change management models currently employed and the effectiveness of their use in the context of healthcare.

Useful websites

www.kingsfund.org.uk/publications/leadership-and-leadership-development-health-care

Link to a report on leadership in healthcare: a summary of the evidence base, outlining the main implications for leadership in healthcare.

www.mindtools.com/cktb5oo/leadership-tools

Mindtool provides a range of learning resources to help you to develop professionally.

www.england.nhs.uk/sustainableimprovement/change-model/

The NHS Change model was developed in 2012; here you will find an overview of this framework.

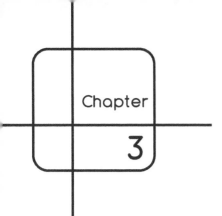

Chapter 3

Understanding interpersonal skills for leadership across multiple settings

Hazel Cowls

NMC STANDARDS OF PROFICIENCY FOR NURSING ASSOCIATE

This chapter will address the following platforms and proficiencies:

Platform 1: Being an accountable professional

1.1   understand and act in accordance with the Code: Professional standards of practice and behaviour for nurses, midwives and nursing associates, and fulfil all registration requirements.

Platform 4: Working in teams

4.1   demonstrate an awareness of the roles, responsibilities and scope of practice of different members of the nursing and interdisciplinary team, and their own role within it.

4.2   demonstrate an ability to support and motivate other members of the care team and interact confidently with them.

4.7   support, supervise and act as a role model to nursing associate students, health care support workers and those new to care roles, review the quality of the care they provide, promoting reflection and providing constructive feedback.

Platform 6: Contributing to integrated care

6.1   understand the roles of the different providers of health and care. Demonstrate the ability to work collaboratively and in partnership with professionals from different agencies in interdisciplinary teams.

Annexe A: Communication and relationship management skills

At the point of registration, the nursing associate will be able to safely demonstrate the following skills:

4.   Demonstrate effective communication skills for working in professional teams.

Introduction

In Chapter 1 you considered the influence of policy and political drivers that impact health and care provision. You are aware that health and social care provision to patients in our communities are delivered by a wider team of professionals that coordinate roles and responsibilities to ensure patients receive personalised high-quality care. Often voluntary and community services are working in conjunction with health and social care professionals to provide additional services such as a mental health charity delivering a well-being café; a local group running a dementia café or a library running a book club. The benefits of including other agencies to support healthcare are that it will reduce the overall burden on the NHS and may also lead to people having access to services within their communities. Regardless of who is delivering care, the patient, carer and other service users' experience is a key concern for everyone delivering care – whether this is in primary, secondary or private and voluntary sector.

The role of the nursing associate is to bridge the gap between healthcare assistants and registered nurses (RCN, n.d.). In this chapter, you will explore the interpersonal skills that will enable you to lead, support and motivate other members of the care team and interact confidently with them to deliver safe patient care (NMC, 2018b). You will explore the importance of leading others and of followership, as well as recognising the value of interdisciplinary team-working. Finally, you will consider how to develop your own leadership knowledge and skills within your role.

Leadership skills

You probably understand that the application of leadership theory in practice largely depends upon the situation. For example, if an immediate change in practice is required due to a severe clinical incident, then the leader/manager is likely to adopt an authoritarian approach to leadership (see Chapter 2). Whereas if the leader is considering introducing a new piece of equipment into practice, the leader is more likely to adopt a democratic leadership style. Regardless of the situation, the way in which we communicate and manage ourselves is central to being an effective leader and follower. Therefore, we need to recognise our personal qualities, our strengths and limitations to develop our leadership and interpersonal skills so that we can communicate effectively with other people.

The words 'leader' and 'manager' are often used synonymously, but the two roles are quite different. A manager has designated authority and will communicate clearly with the team providing structure, establishing rules, organising staffing, budgets, resource planning and problem-solving. In contrast, a leader does not need to be a person of authority, but a leader may be knowledgeable and will be able to demonstrate interpersonal skills such as listening, coaching and motivating others (Kotter, 1990). If we think about the skills that we would like to see in a leader we would probably come up with a similar list:

- active listening;
- empathy;
- able to share ideas;
- clear strategic thinking;
- flexible;
- approachable;
- creative and visionary;
- good time management.

You may have noticed that this list appears to focus on the *soft skills* or interpersonal skills between a leader and others. In Chapter 2, you may recall that participative and relationship theory also focus on these skills and the connections with others.

In 2013, the NHS Leadership Academy developed the Healthcare Leadership model. The model is an evidence-based research model that reflects the values of people working in the NHS, what people know about effective leadership, so drawing on earlier work, and what the public are asking from healthcare professionals (Storey and Holti, 2013). The aim of this model is to help people understand how their leadership behaviours can affect the culture and climate that you and your colleagues work in. The leadership model is for everyone, not just those that are in formal leadership roles, and is made up of nine dimensions (see Figure 3.1). Although the model recognises the importance of personal qualities, these are not highlighted separately but are threaded throughout the nine dimensions.

Activity 3.1   Research

Review the nine dimensions in the *Healthcare Leadership Model* (2013) document (available at: www.leadershipacademy.nhs.uk/wp-content/uploads/2014/10/NHSLeadership-LeadershipModel-colour.pdf). A brief description of each dimension is given, with behaviours shown as part of a four-part scale ranging from essential to proficient, strong and exemplary.

- Are there any areas that you are demonstrating exemplary practice?
- How are you demonstrating this practice?
- Are there any areas that you are demonstrating essential practice and how will you develop your skills and practice?

An outline answer is given to this activity at the end of the chapter.

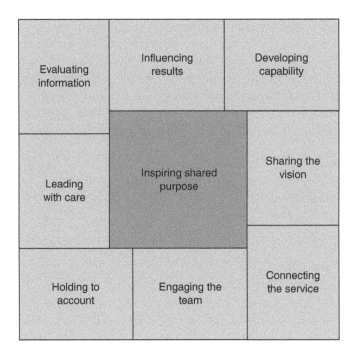

Figure 3.1 NHS Healthcare Leadership model, which demonstrates the behaviours expected of all staff involved in healthcare

Source: Adapted from the NHS Leadership Academy (2013).

Leading others and followership

Most academic literature focuses on leadership and team-working in the healthcare setting but there is also evidence that the followership role is equally important, especially as followers represent around 80 per cent of the workforce (Crawford and Daniels, 2014). This section will explore leadership, team-working and followership. Healthcare teams are a group of individuals working together to achieve a common goal, each possessing different skills and expertise that can be drawn on to deliver evidence-based care. The team leader is a person who may be responsible for ensuring that the goal is achieved. Sometimes this may be the manager but not always, as the manager may allocate leadership to someone with leadership skills to motivate others to achieve the goal. A good team leader has many attributes, including:

- knowing individual members of the team;
- knowing individual members' skills and capabilities;
- being a good communicator and being empathetic to individuals within the team;
- being knowledgeable but also recognising their own limitations;
- being able to act as a positive role model;
- acting with professionalism;
- being assertive;
- delegating tasks appropriately (see Chapter 6).

Interestingly, this list focuses on interpersonal skills rather than clinical expertise. That does not mean we do not expect leaders to be experts; rather we may look for other attributes in a leader. This may include feeling supported, valued and having a feeling of belonging and safety. You may have noticed that many of these attributes would also require a leader to be compassionate.

In recent years there has been more written about compassionate leadership and a recent definition of a compassionate leader is a person who 'seeks to ensure that everyone has and feels responsibility for leading in service of the communities cared for by health and social care' (West, 2021, p. 155). But compassionate leadership is not new; one survey asked participants to state the top ten characteristics of a compassionate leader. The top ten responses were:

1. emotional intelligence
2. integrity
3. listening
4. trust
5. authenticity
6. openness
7. caring
8. reflectiveness
9. commitment
10. genuineness (NHS England, 2014).

Poorkavoos (2016) carried out a survey to understand compassion in the workplace and collected 554 responses from employees of different backgrounds and levels of management. The results of the survey concluded that a compassionate leader has five key attributes which are: being present; understanding the challenges that colleagues face; listening to colleagues' concerns or fears; and being non-judgemental and empathetic, where necessary taking appropriate action to support colleagues.

Some people may view compassionate leadership as a soft and ineffective leadership approach, but recently we have seen a growth in compassionate leadership where organisations have altered as people develop different ways of working (West, 2021). It has become increasingly important for individuals and leaders to develop their interpersonal skills. In fact, it has been suggested that compassion is a fundamental nursing value that has become increasingly important since the Covid-19 pandemic (Vogel and Flint, 2021). West (2021), in his work around compassionate leadership, stated that the skills of a compassionate leader are simply demonstrated in the leader by:

- *attending*: listening to the person;
- *understanding*: taking time to understand how another person is feeling;
- *empathising*: showing genuine warmth and being empathic;
- *helping*: helping people practically and taking time to deal with any problem presented.

As shown, there is wide evidence to suggest that compassionate leadership can result in better support for staff and patient care. In Chapter 8, you will read about compassionate leadership and understand how compassionate leaders support, provide feedback, supervise and act as a role model.

But to be an effective leader we also need followers: 'Without followers there cannot be leaders and without leaders there cannot be followers' (Barr and Dowding, 2019). Followership is difficult to define as it does depend on the situation, the leader and the followers. The concept of followership has been described as the 'flipside of leadership' (Hersey et al., 1996). Kelley (1992) described a followership matrix and identified five types of followers.

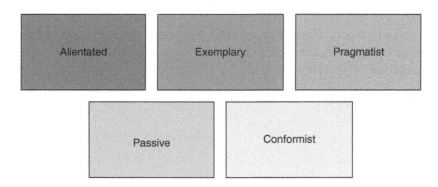

Figure 3.2   Five types of followers

Source: Adapted from Kelley, 1992.

Kelley (1992) went on to explain that there are two dimensions to followership: engaged and critical thinkers. A person who is actively engaged will question and drive forward change or a task. In contrast, a person who is passively engaged will wait for direction from the leader or manager. Followers are also either independent or dependent critical thinkers. An independent critical thinker can manage themselves, reflect on their practice, develop their skills and analyse the consequences of any actions (Northouse, 2019). For example, an exemplary follower and a conformist follower are both active followers, but an exemplary follower is more likely to question, or lead compared with a conformist follower who will follow instructions. The characteristics of each type of follower are listed in Table 3.1.

Table 3.1   Characteristics of followers

Follower	Skills
Exemplary	Confident, good communicator, critical thinker, able to challenge the leader if necessary. Exemplary followers cope with change well, often putting their own views forward. Kelley called this group 'The Stars'.
Conformist	Active doers that will follow leaders' directions but do not challenge or question any instructions. They are loyal and will avoid any conflict. Kelley called this group 'The Yes-People'.
Passive	Unquestionably follow the leader and wait for further directions. This follower tends not to show any initiative and is susceptible to being micromanaged. Kelley called this group 'The Sheep'.
Alienated	Independent critical thinkers who will proactively supply alternative solutions. This follower can be viewed as cynical and negative.
Pragmatist	Possess a moderate level of engagement and moderate level of critical thinking, so tend to support the status quo before making any decisions. Kelley called this group 'The Survivor'.

Activity 3.2   Reflection

- As a trainee nursing associate (TNA), can you think of a time when you have been a follower?
- Which type of follower were you?
- Why do you think you are that type of follower?
- Do you think your followership behaviours are constant all the time?

As this activity is based on your own observation, there is no outline answer at the end of the chapter.

You may recall times in your career or study that you have acted as a passive follower, maybe when you began a new placement, joined a new team or began a new role. However, as you develop your knowledge and skills you may have acted as a pragmatist or as an exemplary follower, questioning or developing practice.

The following case study illustrates the leader and different types of followers.

Case study: Temi

Temi is a second-year TNA working in a GP practice. The practice manager has suggested that Temi can run their own NHS well-being clinic. Temi is enthusiastic about this and meets their practice assessor to discuss how they can prepare for the clinic. The practice assessor is supportive and recommends that Temi read relevant documents on NHS Health Checks and Making Every Contact Count (MECC). However, during a coffee break Temi overhears Colleague A saying: *'Well, I don't know why they are running the clinic as they do not even have access to the online consultation pages.'* Colleague B states: *'I think it will be good for their development, I suppose Temi just needs to make sure they can access the consultation page.'*

This short case study illustrates the leader and different types of followers. The practice manager is the leader and is supported by Temi's practice assessor (PA) who is acting as an exemplary follower as the PA is passing on instructions but also making recommendations. Temi is also an active follower but rather than questioning, they are following instructions and this would be right at this time, so Temi is a conformist follower. Unfortunately, not everyone is supportive of the plan. Colleague A appears to be critical, questioning the plan and looking for reasons why this would not work. This behaviour suggests that Colleague A is acting as an alienated follower. Meanwhile Colleague B is more cautious and may be avoiding any conflict by acknowledging Colleague A's concern but also raising a positive. Colleague B is acting as a pragmatic follower.

Activity 3.3   Critical thinking

Leaders need to take different approaches/use different skills to communicate with and motivate different types of followers. What interpersonal skills would you need to demonstrate when communicating with colleagues who are:

1. an exemplary follower?
2. a passive follower?
3. an alienated follower?

An outline answer is given to this activity at the end of the chapter.

In summary, you could argue that many professionals working in teams across health and social care are followers as we work in teams to plan and deliver care, attend team meetings, demonstrate different technology or equipment being used in practice. A good leader will create an environment that is conducive to developing followers such as leading by example, welcoming questions from the team, seeking feedback from members of their team, delegating responsibly (see Chapter 6) and utilising expertise within their team (Smith-Trudeau, 2017). But followership is not just about people who follow in teams; it is also about the relationship with members of the team and the leader. In fact, followership is viewed as a relationship role where followers may influence the leader and contribute to organisational goals; leaders cannot function without followers (Stanley, 2017).

Understanding team-working

A TNA is a member of a wider team working across health and social care sectors and as a new member of the team you may come across a range of terms that are used to explain team-working. Terms that have been used when explaining team-working for health and social care professionals include: *multidisciplinary, multiprofessional, multiagency, interdisciplinary, interprofessional* and *collaborative*. But if we look at the meaning of the prefixes used in these words they are:

inter- used to form an adjective meaning between or among people, things or places

multi- means many

Mumma and Nelson (2008) differentiated between the terms *multidisciplinary, interprofessional* and *transdisciplinary*:

*   *multidisciplinary* – there are clear boundaries between disciplines and discipline-specific goals;
*   *interprofessional* – work collaboratively to identify patient goals and work beyond discipline-specific work;

- *transdisciplinary* – work flexibly to minimise duplication of work and therefore boundaries across disciplines are blurred.

However, NHS England (2014) described multidisciplinary as working with many disciplines utilising their experience and knowledge and that a *multidisciplinary approach* enables multiple disciplines to explore problems outside normal professional boundaries and to reach solutions based on a new understanding of each situation. This description implies that disciplines can work outside their normal boundaries.

In summary, it appears that the words are interchangeable with *interdisciplinary* meaning cross-disciplinary, multidisciplinary, cross-practice or collaborative (*Cambridge English Dictionary*, 2022). In clinical practice, an interdisciplinary team includes professionals from many disciplines who work collaboratively with the patient and each other to assess, plan and deliver care. An example of this could be a trauma team working in the emergency department looking after a person who has been in a road traffic accident. The team may consist of a medical clinician, radiographer, plaster technician, nurses and ancillary workers, and will also include people outside the department such as a biochemist, theatre staff, critical care unit and bed coordinators.

Activity 3.4   Reflection

Thinking about interdisciplinary team-working, please reflect on a time when you have worked effectively as a member of the interdisciplinary team.

As this activity is based on your own observation, there is no outline answer at the end of the chapter.

Activity 3.5   Reflection

As a TNA, you will have personal experience of working in a new role or beginning a new course and needing to explain to others:

- why you are studying;
- what you will gain from study;
- how that will improve your practice or your patient care;
- and how your role is different from a Level 2 registered nurse role or an assistant practitioner role.

For this activity, please consider the interpersonal skills that you have used/or may use to answer any of the questions above.

As this activity is based on your own observation, there is no outline answer at the end of the chapter.

It is important that we recognise what makes an effective team, as well as the potential barriers to team-working. Team-working has been discussed in many leadership journals and books and the consensus is that good team-working will lead to good patient care. However, the creation of an effective team is not something that occurs overnight; it requires effort not only from the organisation, but also from leaders and individuals within the team. Established teams usually fall into three basic sets:

- *high-performance teams* – these teams have an established and clear purpose, are committed, with a sense of ownership of the team, organisational goals and values;
- *functional teams* – these teams work well together but lack confidence to develop and there is a hierarchy within the team;
- *struggling teams* – these teams are not committed to working together, they do not meet and avoid any team discussions (Stanley, 2017).

The goal for most teams is to be a functional or high-performance team. The factors that influence how people work together are the team dynamics such as individual characteristics, individual roles, level of education and lines of management. One theorist suggested that all teams go through stages of development, from a newly formed group to a functioning team (Tuckman, 1965). The initial model included four stages, but following a systematic review (Tuckman and Jenson, 1977) the fifth stage, adjourning/mourning was included.

Table 3.2 How a team develops

Development stage	Brief details
Forming	Initial meeting of the group, getting to know individual members, orientation phase, limited or no structure at this stage.
Storming	Individuals and group explore the purpose of the group; this may include questioning, some disagreement, conflicts.
Norming	Agreement on group objectives, roles allocated/offered, ground rules are agreed.
Performing	Regular group meetings to review progress, highlighting any issues and planning.
Adjourning/ Mourning	On completion of group task, the group disband but may arrange follow-up meeting after summative evaluation.

Source: Tuckman, 1965.

Although Tuckman's theory is well known, the Affina Team Performance Inventory (ATPI) has been developed to measure teams' potential to perform effectively (West et al., 2004). Like the NHS Leadership model (2013), the ATPI assessment is available online and measures three specific elements that are essential for team-working: team inputs + processes = team outputs; these lead to effective team-working and performance.

Understanding the theory: ATPI assessment of team effectiveness

Team inputs – focuses on how the organisation leads and manages change, communicates with employees and ensures that there are adequate support and resources available to ensure staff are competent.

Processes – focuses on the processes that relate to leading, managing and coaching teams to achieve a goal.

Team outputs – relates to team member satisfaction, how the team's will communicate with each other. Ensuring staff will be supportive and able to manage their own and other's emotions. Ensuring staff will work cohesively to achieve a common goal and will problem-solve and work with others to reduce any conflict or misunderstandings.

These elements can be applied to any environment in health and social care, but a good example of an effective team in clinical practice is the in-hospital cardiac arrest team, as they are a team of professionals working together to achieve a common goal or purpose. The following elements and dimensions of a good resuscitation team are:

- *Team inputs*

The organisation communicates openly with employees and provides a clear Trust Policy on Cardiac Resuscitation. The organisation will provide relevant training to ensure staff are competent. The team will debrief after any clinical emergency.

- *Processes*

Individuals in the resuscitation team will usually have complementary skills and with skilled leadership will work together to achieve a goal. The team will work best if they know each other's name and skill set. Some organisations recommend that the resuscitation team meet at the beginning of the day for a briefing.

- *Team outputs*

The resuscitation team will be accountable for their own and the team's actions, they will communicate openly with each other and provide feedback or suggest different ways of working. The team will be supportive of each other and enable others to achieve their best.

Tuckman (1965) and West et al. (2004) have explored the process of effective team-working; understanding how individuals work within a team is as important as understanding how teams function. Belbin's work (2000) looked specifically at the roles of individuals within teams. Belbin (2000) recognised that high-performing teams are made up of a mixture of individuals with different qualities and attributes. The advantage to having individuals with different skills and attributes is that the leader and team can draw on individual strengths. Belbin (2000) concluded that if we all work similarly then this may be counter-productive, whereas if we question and challenge the status quo then this will lead to innovation and change. Table 3.3 illustrates details of each team role; you will note that the nine roles are separated into three specific workplace orientations. People-orientated roles focus on the relationship with the team, thinking-orientated roles focus on what individuals bring to the team and, finally, action-orientated roles focus on the actions of individuals.

Table 3.3 Individual team roles and workplace orientation

Individual team role	Attributes	Workplace orientation
Resource investigator	Uses their inquisitive nature to find ideas to bring back to the team	*People- orientated roles*
Team-worker	Helps the team to gel and ensures tasks are completed	
Coordinator	Focuses on team objectives and delegates work appropriately	
Monitor-evaluator	Provides a logical eye, weighs up the team's options in a dispassionate way	*Thinking-orientated roles*
Plant	Highly creative and good at probem-solving	
Specialist	Brings in-depth knowledge	
Shaper	Thrives on pressure and needed to drive the team forward	*Action-orientated roles*
Implementor	Needed for planning and strategy	
Complete finisher	Used at the end of tasks to review	

According to Belbin (2000) everyone will bring specific skills to the team, with some people having more than one role within the team. Below are the strengths and weaknesses of the team roles.

Table 3.4 Strengths and weaknesses of individual team roles

Team role	Strengths	Weaknesses
Resource investigator	Uses their inquisitive nature to find ideas to bring back to the team	Over optimistic, loses interest
Team-worker	Cooperative, diplomatic	Indecisive, avoids conflict
Coordinator	Confident, decision-maker, delegates	May be intolerant of people who take time to make decisions

Team role	Strengths	Weaknesses
Monitor-evaluator	Strategic, discerning, sees all options	Can lack drive and be over critical
Plant	Creative, imaginative, problem-solver	Too preoccupied to communicate effectively
Specialist	Provides specialist knowledge, single-minded and dedicated	'Tunnel-visioned'
Shaper	Challenging and dynamic, driven	Prone to provocation and may offend
Implementor	Practical, reliable and efficient	Can be inflexible
Complete finisher	Conscientious, polishes and perfects work	Can be anxious and reluctant to delegate

Team-working is more than understanding how teams form and the attributes of individual team members; it is also about the cognitive, social and personal skills of individuals within the team. Let's refer to the cardiac arrest team, mentioned previously. This team will need to have advanced clinical skills (technical) and each member of the team also needs to have non-technical skills. The non-technical skills include situational awareness, decision-making, team-working and task management and these skills complement the technical skills, leading to safe and effective care (Resuscitation Council, 2021). An explanation of each of the non-technical skills is below.

- *Situational awareness* is having an awareness of the environment and the current situation.
- *Decision-making* is the cognitive process of choosing a particular course of action. Decision-making can be undertaken by an individual or as a team.
- *Team-working* and *leadership* are about people working together to achieve a goal and require effective communication, active listening, being accountable, being competent and committed to the goal/tasks.
- *Task management* is ensuring all staff are aware of the tasks that need to be completed, taking into consideration any time scales to complete the task, what specific skills are needed to complete the task and who is available to complete the task.

The key non-technical skills could also apply to other clinical settings and situations. The two scenarios that follow will illustrate these non-technical skills.

Case study: Aiden

Aiden is a second-year TNA and is working on an elder care ward. One of the elderly gentlemen on the ward has tested positive for Covid-19 and needs to be isolated at once but a patient transfer ambulance has just arrived with two patients who need to

(Continued)

(Continued)

be admitted to the ward. Aiden liaises with the registered nurse (RN) and a year one TNA. The team decide that the RN takes a 'handover' of care from the ambulance drivers while Aiden and the TNA move the elderly gentleman who has tested Covid-positive into a side room. The RN requests that Aiden reports back once he has completed that task and then he can supervise the TNA admitting one of the new patients.

This case study is a good example of team-working together. The team is aware of the current situation and works together to decide on a plan of action, with specific tasks being allocated to members of the team. The decision-making and task allocation in this scenario appears to be quite simple as the team is working together to achieve a common goal.

Case study: Martha

Martha is a TNA working in adult health but in order to gain cross-field experience Martha has been allocated to an acute community mental health unit. Martha is excited to join the placement as she has never worked in mental health. On day one Martha meets Catalina, a 26-year-old woman who was admitted to the unit two months earlier. Catalina lives with her mother and three-year-old daughter in a two-bedroomed house. Catalina does not work as she is a full-time mother. Catalina is from Portugal and does not speak English. Catalina was admitted to the unit following attempted suicide and she presented with a deep ligature wound to her neck. Martha noticed that Catalina rarely left her room and did not engage with any other residents or staff. As a TNA working in adult health Martha felt competent at changing Catalina's wound dressing and during this time tried to communicate with Catalina by speaking in Spanish. This surprised Catalina and she did respond to Martha.

Martha spoke to her PA and requested that she led in Catalina's care as she felt she was developing a therapeutic relationship with Catalina. Over the coming weeks Catalina continued to engage with Martha, leaving her room to sit with Martha at lunchtime and starting to join other patients. Martha attends multidisciplinary (MDT) meetings and acts as an advocate for Catalina.

This case study illustrates the importance of working in an interdisciplinary team to achieve a goal. Martha is confident and able to develop a therapeutic relationship with Catalina and work with the team. Martha has demonstrated good non-technical skills such as situation awareness, decision-making and team-working and is acting as an advocate for Catalina by being able to attend MDT meetings and communicating back to Catalina.

Developing your own leadership style

You are probably wondering how you can develop your own leadership style and interpersonal skills as a TNA and on becoming an RNA. In this section, you will be asked to complete some activities to assess your own leadership style. As a pre-registration professional, there are three stages of developing as a leader.

1. *Focus on self*: by developing your self-awareness, self-efficacy to understand your own beliefs, attitudes, values, knowledge, attributes and skills to develop your own leadership behaviours.
2. *Working with others*: develop your interpersonal skills to connect with a diverse range of people across organisations and develop your team-working skills.
3. *Improving healthcare*: develop and lead teams to make a positive change in practice ensuring high-quality, safe patient care (HEE, 2018).

Kouzes and Posner (2011) suggested that self-discovery and self-awareness are critical to developing the capacity to lead and this can be achieved through reflective practice. Furthermore, our ability to lead others is based on our own values and beliefs (Kouzes and Posner, 2013) – for example, how can we lead if we do not have any strong values or beliefs. As you develop your leadership skills you may want to consider how you see yourself and how others see you as a leader. It is important to attain feedback from others as we are not always aware of how other people may see us. The Johari Window (Luft and Ingham, 1955) allows us to view how we see ourselves and how we are viewed. The window has four areas as shown in Figure 3.3.

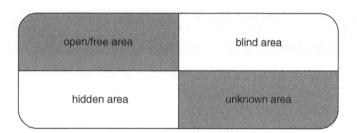

Figure 3.3 Johari Window self-awareness framework

Source: Adapted from Luft and Ingham (1955), p. 10, as in Ellis (2022).

The relevance of this model is that it can be beneficial to team meetings to analyse decision-making situations, raising awareness of how others perceive us, or even the qualities that we have but are not aware of – all of which can add to information so that decisions can be made. The model can also be used for analysing problem-solving and conflict management situations (Gopee and Galloway, 2017).

The Healthcare Leadership model suggests that other personal qualities such as self-confidence, self-knowledge and resilience influence how we behave and are especially important when we are working in teams. It is important to be aware of our strengths and limitations in each of these areas as this will have an impact on the team you work alongside as well as the organisation (NHS Leadership Academy, 2013).

As a TNA who will be acting as a leader in clinical practice you will also need to manage your own emotions as well as others. In the context of leadership and management, emotional intelligence (EI) is the ability to recognise and manage emotions, understanding the impact individual emotions may have on decision-making. Often people that are emotionally intelligent can identify their feelings and will carefully consider their actions first before making a decision. As a TNA you will need to be aware of other people's emotions and ensure that decisions made will not impact negatively on patient care.

As a TNA you will need to continually develop your own personal resilience as you strive to be an accountable practitioner. But what does that mean? The word 'resilience' is derived from the Latin word *resilia*, meaning the 'the ability of people or things to recover quickly after something unpleasant, such as shock, injury' (*Oxford Learner's Dictionary*, n.d.) or, put another way, that it is having the ability to return to a state of normality or to 'bounce back' from adversity or trauma and remain focused and optimistic about the future (Dyer and McGuinness, 1996).

Take a moment to think about what helps you to 'bounce back' or cope with the stressors being placed on you. You may have considered internal factors such as your ability to be adaptable, developing your confidence. External factors could include social support around you. You may have thought about self-compassion as this is positively related to resilience, engagement, intrinsic motivation and well-being with resilience being identified as predictors of self-compassion (Kotera et al., 2021).

The following activities will help you to develop your leadership style but, remember, developing your practice is a continual process.

Activity 3.6　　Reflection

As discussed, self-discovery and self-awareness are important as you develop your leadership style. The Healthcare Leadership model's self-assessment tool will encourage you to think about the dimensions of the Healthcare Leadership model that are particularly important to you and will help you to compare how you rate yourself in these dimensions to inform your development plans. Please complete the *Healthcare Leadership model self-assessment tool* available at NHS Leadership Academy. You will need to register for a free NHS Leadership Academy ID on NHSx. Once you have completed your self-assessment, please download the results.

Consider the following:

1.　What are your strengths?
2.　Which areas do you need to develop?
3.　How will you develop specific areas?

As this activity is based on your own observation, there is no outline answer at the end of the chapter.

Another way of looking at your leadership and interpersonal skills is to complete a SWOT analysis (Strengths, Weakness, Opportunities and Threats). Developed by Andrews (1971), this framework was originally used in business to assess a company's strategic position in business. However, this approach could also be used in healthcare by teams to assess what they do well and areas that they can improve or by individuals as part of their annual performance review. The strengths and weaknesses are internal factors, while opportunities and threats are usually external to the individual or team. There are five steps to conducting a SWOT analysis:

1. Step 1. List all your or your teams' strengths.
2. Step 2. List all your or your teams' weaknesses.
3. Step 3. List all the opportunities for the future and these will become your strengths.
4. Step 4. List all the threats for the future and these will become your weaknesses.
5. Step 5. Review your SWOT and develop a plan of action to address each area of the SWOT analysis.

Some people prefer to use the acronym SCOT analysis which stands for Strengths, Challenges, Opportunities and Threats as it may be viewed less negatively, replacing weakness with a challenge. However, like SWOT, applying this process will enable individuals or organisations to leverage their strengths, understand any challenges or weaknesses, recognise any opportunities and counteract any threats.

As a TNA, can you see how this framework may help you to develop your leadership and interpersonal skills? For example, you may have identified that you have some of the necessary skills and attributes of a leader, but you recognise that a challenge is that your role is a relatively new role and not well understood by colleagues. However, your manager is supportive of your role and encourages you to speak to the team about your role.

The next step to developing your leadership skills is to consider your goals and develop an action plan. There are several acronyms and models that can help you to develop your goals and action plan. SMART is an acronym that can be used as a guide for setting goals.

- *Specific* – is your goal clear? For example, what do you want to achieve, who is involved, where is the location?
- *Measurable* – can you measure your goal? How will you know when you have achieved your goal?
- *Achievable* – is your goal realistic and attainable. How will you carry out this goal, what do you need?
- *Relevant* – is this goal important to you? Is it the right time?
- *Time bound* – every goal needs a target date as a focus.

SMART is a well-established tool that can help you to create a clear and meaningful goal. The first example does not fit the SMART rules and therefore the person is less likely to achieve their goal. Whereas the SMART goal is clear, measurable, achievable, relevant and time bound.

Simple Goal Example = I want to get fit.

SMART goal example = I am going to follow the Couch to 10K (C210K) app training programme weekly to run the local 10K in six months from now.

An alternative model to SMART is the GROW model. This is a four-stage coaching and goal-setting model (Whitmore, 2017) and can be used to coach yourself and others. The acronym GROW stands for:

- **G**oal – what do you want?
- **R**eality – where are you now?
- **O**ptions – what could you do?
- **W**ill – what will you do?

If we apply the same goal to this model it would look like this:

- **G**oal – I want to get fit and run the local 10K in six months from now.
- **R**eality – I am not very active and therefore need to pace and plan my exercise regime.
- **O**ptions – I am motivated and can plan my day to include a walk and run each day. The C210K app is available for free; I can download this to my mobile phone. This means I can follow the instructions while I am exercising.
- **W**ill – I plan to follow the C210K training programme via the app. I will run weekly and build up my activity each week.

Chapter summary

This chapter has explored the interpersonal skills that lead to good leadership and team-working. A positive leadership style may lead to satisfied, loyal and engaged employees; high-quality, safe and compassionate care; increased service user satisfaction; and a successful healthcare organisation (NHS Leadership Academy, 2013). The literature suggests that organisations need leaders as well as followers and that being a follower is not subservient to a leader. There are five types of followership: exemplary, conformist, pragmatist, alienated and passive and, depending upon the situation, people can move through different followership styles. This chapter has also presented various tools that will enable you to develop your own leadership style and resilience such as SWOT/SCOT analysis, SMART goals, GROW.

Activities: brief outline answers

Activity 3.1

The aim of this activity is to understand the Healthcare Leadership model as this model is widely referred to in clinical practice and you will be completing a self-assessment for a later activity.

Activity 3.3

- An exemplary follower is engaged, motivated and an independent critical thinker. A leader would want to be encouraging to an exemplary follower, to listen to their ideas and to be supportive so that they can develop their skills.
- A passive follower is supportive of the leader, may feel underconfident and may seek support and regular feedback; this follower will not challenge the leader. The leader will need to understand that a passive follower will require clear instructions.
- An alienated follower is an independent critical thinker but can also be passive and critical of any decision-making. The leader may need to manage difficult conversations and conflict which can be achieved through effective communication skills such as active listening, paraphrasing, understanding the follower's point of view.

Further reading

NHS Leadership Academy learning hub. Available at: learninghub.leadership academy.nhs.uk /all-bitesize/

This is a series of short courses to help you to build your knowledge and skills. The bitesize learning will cover topics such as leadership, team-working and resilience. You will need to register and log in to access the free resources.

NHS England (2014) *MDT Development: Working Toward an Effective Multidisciplinary/Multiagency Team*. Available at: www.england.nhs.uk/wp-content/uploads/2015/01/mdt-dev-guid-flat-fin.pdf

This document provides teams with a non-judgemental set of tools that can be used to self-assess their teams and benchmark against descriptions of team-working.

Royal College of Physicians (2021) *Modern Ward Rounds: Good Practice for Multidisciplinary Review*. Available at: www.rcplondon.ac.uk/projects/outputs/modern-ward-rounds

The guide brings together examples of best practice for modern ward rounds, enabling individuals and clinical teams to self-assess against this and identify areas for improvement in their own clinical practice.

Useful websites

www.belbin.com/about/belbin-team-roles

Belbin Team Roles defines 'team role' as one of nine clusters of behavioural attributes.

www.leadershipacademy.nhs.uk/resources/healthcare-leadership-model/

The Healthcare Leadership model is useful for everyone because it describes the things you can see leaders doing at work and how you can develop as a leader, even if you're not in a formal leadership role. The leadership model is made up of nine leadership dimensions and you can explore each of these dimensions.

http://leadershipacademy.nhs.uk/resources/healthcare-leadership-model/ supporting-tools-resources/healthcare-leadership-model-self-assessment- tool/

Self-assessment will help you to understand your own leadership behaviours and highlight areas of strength, as well as areas that you may need greater focus on.

www.kingsfund.org.uk/topics/clinical-leadership

The King's Fund is an independent charitable organisation working to improve health and social care in England. A priority of the King's Fund is to support people and leaders working in health and social care.

www.kingsfund.org.uk/audio-video/podcast

The King's Fund Podcast talks with experts from the King's Fund and beyond about all things related to health and social care and leadership. New episodes each month.

https://jenniferjacksonrn.org/resilience/resilience-in-systems/

The Resilience Challenge game. The idea for this game is to introduce new ideas about patient safety to clinicians. You will be guided through a patient journey and will need to make choices for each scenario. You will receive feedback on your choices and consider how these impact on patient care.

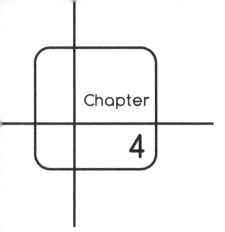

Understanding and applying the principles of human and environmental factors in relation to leadership

Sarah Tobin

NMC STANDARDS OF PROFICIENCY FOR NURSING ASSOCIATE

This chapter will address the following platforms and proficiencies:

Platform 1: Being an accountable professional

1.2 understand and apply relevant legal, regulatory and governance requirements, policies, and ethical frameworks, including any mandatory reporting duties, to all areas of practice.

1.5 understand the demands of professional practice and demonstrate how to recognise signs of vulnerability in themselves or their colleagues and the action required to minimise risks to health.

1.8 understand and explain the meaning of resilience and emotional intelligence, and their influence on an individual's ability to provide care.

1.10 demonstrate the skills and abilities required to develop, manage and maintain appropriate relationships with people, their families, carers and colleagues.

1.12 recognise and report any factors that may adversely impact safe and effective care provision.

Platform 4: Working in teams

4.3 understand and apply the principles of human factors and environmental factors when working in teams.

Platform 5: Improving safety and quality of care

5.1 understand and apply the principles of health and safety legislation and regulations and maintain safe work and care environments.

> # Chapter aims
>
> After reading this chapter you will be able to:
>
> - explain terms such as human factors and emotional intelligence and understand the wider meaning of the term *environment*;
> - identify the importance of non-technical skills;
> - develop an understanding of situational awareness and how decisions are made;
> - explore how your leadership skills can contribute to patient safety and environmental culture.

Introduction

This chapter will explain what human and environmental factors are, and explore how these can impact your practice, leadership and, ultimately, patient care. It would seem logical that if you intend to lead (or be a useful follower), understanding the people you work with and what may motivate or impede your work would be useful. Equally, the influence of the environment on you, your colleagues and therefore the patient can help inform and improve your understanding of how care is, and can be, led.

As previously discussed in Chapters 1 and 2, nursing associates (NAs) may believe that they have a limited leadership role or that leadership is the preserve of those with managerial roles. The RCN describes the concept of *collective leadership*, which is an assumption that leadership can and should be provided by anybody (2022a). And, while the NMC Standards (2018c) do not specifically describe the requirements to be a leader, they do make it clear that aspects of leadership such as supervision, delegation, providing feedback, self-management and acting as a role model are part of the role requirements. All these elements – elements that contribute to more effective patient care – can and will be influenced by both human and environmental factors.

Nearly 60 per cent of the staff employed by the NHS in 2021 were qualified clinical staff (doctors, nurses and midwives, scientific, therapeutic and technical staff, and ambulance staff) (NHS Digital, 2021c). The people who work for the NHS and other health providers are undoubtedly the biggest asset any organisation has, but human beings are ... human! They make mistakes and can be impacted by numerous internal and external factors which might affect their behaviour and performance. Alexander Pope (1688–1744) suggested that 'To err is human: to forgive, divine' (1963), but in healthcare situations where to err can cause devastating consequences it is better to try and reduce the risk of error rather than rely on forgiveness! Effective leadership that considers the needs, strengths and weaknesses of those being led should, in turn, provide a safer, more effective and kinder environment for patients.

Case study: Tina

Tina is an RNA in a community hospital and is on the final night shift of four; she is working with a newly qualified RN and a healthcare assistant (HCA) in a ward for 22 patients. Tina slept badly during the day before coming to work and for the last few days as there are roadworks in the street creating a lot of noise.

Tina and the RN each take responsibility for half of the patients for their drug administration and care management. Tina starts the 10pm drug round and is aware that there are two patients on her 'side' of the unit who have been highlighted as of specific concern. One patient is receiving end of life care in a side room and has several family members who are visiting and who have permission to do so at any time – this patient's condition has significantly deteriorated during the evening. Another patient has dementia, has been getting increasingly agitated and has attempted to leave the ward on several occasions, becoming both verbally and physically aggressive when encouraged to remain.

Tina can see that the HCA is walking with the patent with dementia and trying to convince them to return to their bed, she can see that the situation is challenging, especially as several call bells are also going off. Tina is rushing to dispense the medications for the final patient on the round when a very distressed man comes up to her and states that he believes that his mother in the side room has just died, he is sobbing and obviously very distressed. The RN, who is just completing his drug round, comes past and seeing the situation offers to complete the drug round for Tina so that she can attend to the family in the side room.

Later that night Tina reviews all the drug charts as part of the nightly medication stock take and can see that not only has the RN signed for the medication Tina had dispensed but not administered to the final patient, but he has also signed for the previous patient as well. Tina had given this patient their required medication and realises that she did not sign for it. When she asks the RN, he says that, seeing it unsigned, he assumed it had not been given and so administered the same 10pm medication that Tina had already just given; he reports that the patient did take all of them.

Reading this case study (which is loosely based on a real incident) it is evident that several factors contributed to the drug error that was made, both human and environmental. Not all these factors can be prevented or even anticipated, but many can and should be; by doing so, mistakes, and the subsequent impact for all concerned, can be reduced.

Activity 4.1   Critical thinking

List the factors, either human or environmental, that may have contributed to the drug error that was made. You can make two headings and list them under each one. Then list any relevant NMC Standards of Proficiency that relate to these examples.

An outline answer is provided at the end of this chapter.

Definition and history

Within the Standards (NMC, 2018c, p. 27) the definition of human factors is 'environmental, organisational and job factors, and human and individual characteristics, which influence behaviour at work in a way which can affect health and safety'. The Health and Safety Executive (HSE) (2021) expand on this definition by stating that consideration must be given to how these impact on three connected concepts – the job, the individual and the organisation. The following are examples within each category:

- *The job* – how well a task is defined and explained, workload, the environment including the design of the physical surroundings and the availability and suitability of equipment used; consideration of how possible it is to do the job to the best of the team's ability but also acknowledging weaknesses and limitations.
- *The individual* – their competence, attitude, understanding, level of skill, experience, approach to risk and emotional well-being. Some of these elements are fixed or at least challenging to alter, some may be changed or improved.
- *The organisation* – rotas and shift patterns, culture and emphasis, resource availability and quality, communication and, most definitely, … leadership (at all levels).

Activity 4.2   In practice

Create a table with three headings – see below.

Think of the area where you work; under each heading list as many elements and examples that you can think of that would fit within the category. Use the description above but think of the realities of your experience in practice – one has been provided for you to get you underway.

Table 4.1   The job, the individual, the organisation

The job	The individual	The organisation
A new procedure has been introduced to the unit – it is the first time that you have needed to carry it out.	You are worried about one of your children, you sent them to school despite them saying they felt unwell – you need to phone and check that they are OK.	You have been made aware that you will need to move and work on another ward due to staff shortages.

As this exercise relates to your own work environment no definitive answer has been provided but examples have been included in a generic answer at the end of this chapter.

While the impact of human and environmental factors has always affected patient care, one case served to highlight how significant this impact could be. In 2005 a 37-year-old patient, Elaine Bromiley, was undergoing what should have been a routine surgical procedure. Problems occurred with her airway management and, despite the presence of an experienced and appropriately qualified theatre team and the availability of the emergency equipment that could have saved her life, she died (Reid and Bromiley, 2012). The resultant Harmer inquiry (2010) found that the situation was hampered by a lack of communication between team members and inadequate understanding regarding the use of relevant equipment. Both human and environmental factors had contributed to the tragic death of Elaine, including a failure of leadership and a lack of appreciation of how people react in stressful situations. Elaine's husband was a pilot and campaigned for healthcare organisations to take a similar approach to patient safety as that adopted by the aviation industry, where a history of safety measures and simulated training provision was already embedded. In response, the UK Clinical Human Factors Group was established to include 'a broad coalition of health care professionals, managers, and service users' (Barr and Dowding, 2019, p. 236) to influence the safety agenda across the NHS.

Case study: Jo

Jo is working as an RNA on a busy surgical ward; she has worked there for several years. On the day in question some patients are waiting for surgery, and some have already returned from the morning theatre list. A member of staff called in sick just before the shift and no cover has so far been obtained, despite the nurse-in-charge spending a considerable amount of time in the office phoning possible replacements. Jo is working with a student nurse (St/N), a bank RN and an experienced HCA. Jo has never worked with the RN before and they tell her that this is the first time they have been in this hospital as they only recently moved to the area; they haven't even had an opportunity to undertake the Trust Induction training yet.

Jo becomes increasingly aware that the bank RN is not following what she considers to be appropriate infection control practices – they do not seem to wash their hands very often nor use the alcohol hand gel even when checking wound sites. Jo notices that they seem to be getting frustrated at having to constantly ask where equipment is or how to access notes and information. Jo then overhears the St/N say that they feel the ward is disorganised and that it is hard to work out where things are kept or why colleagues are prioritising one task over another – they say they feel confused and as if they are 'in the way'.

Having read Jo's case study, Activity 4.3 asks you to consider the human and environmental factors in the situation.

Activity 4.3   Reflection

1. What is the risk to patient safety if Jo does nothing?
2. What human and environmental factors have contributed to this situation?
3. How might the Standards help Jo address this situation – which ones are relevant?
4. Take a minute to reflect on how you felt reading this scenario – note your response.

An outline answer has been provided at the end of the chapter.

The importance of non-technical skills

Human and environmental factors influence every element of service provision, so how do nurses and all healthcare workers ensure that they are prepared and capable of addressing these challenges? In recent years greater prominence has been given to the impact and importance of what are called *non-technical skills*; these are the cognitive, social and personal skills that will complement a professional's technical ability (WHO, 2017). This is important when one considers that technical failures are responsible for only a small fraction of adverse events (NHS Scotland, 2010), but failures in non-technical skills are responsible for up to 60 per cent of surgical errors (Gawande et al., 2003) and nearly 98 per cent of medication errors (Gorgich et al., 2016).

According to Flin et al. (2008), non-technical skills can be categorised as relating to three different domains:

- *cognitive*: situational awareness, decision-making;
- *personal*: coping with stress and fatigue, care for self and others;
- *social*: communication, team-working and leadership.

Of course, the distinction between these elements and indeed between technical and non-technical ability is often neither clear cut nor universally relevant. For example, communication is arguably a key *technical* skill and, in some disciplines (mental health nursing, for instance) represents the mechanism necessary to undertake effective assessments and deliver treatment. It can be argued that drawing a distinction between non-technical and technical skills is unhelpful and that effective patient care is provided via a dynamic and complex interplay of knowledge, technical ability and non-technical competence. Yet, it is only in recent years that this interrelatedness has been acknowledged and that human factors education has become more widespread.

Activity 4.4   Critical thinking

Watch the video *The Human Factor: Learning from Gina's Story*, following this link: www.youtube.com/watch?v=IJfoLvLLoFo

Take some time to reflect on what human and environmental factors contributed to what happened to Gina.

In terms of human factors, what failures in non-technical skills can you identify?

An outline answer has been provided at the end of the chapter.

Understanding the theory: the Swiss Cheese model

What happened to Gina had devastating consequences for her and her family; the staff involved were also significantly affected. A human factors model that can be used to help understand why events such as these happen is the 'Swiss Cheese model' developed by psychologist Dr James Reason in 1990. This model suggests that in every system there are many levels of defence that exist to prevent accidents happening. Examples you may be familiar with include checking patient identity details, marking a surgical site prior to surgery, asking a patient if they have any allergies, ensuring equipment has been regularly serviced and so on. Each of the levels of defence can have small 'holes' in it caused by factors such as poor design, organisational decision-making, lack of training, lack or resources and even a procedure itself. These holes are known as either *latent conditions* or *active errors* and can occur and resolve randomly, creating a pattern similar to the holes in a Swiss cheese. If, for whatever reason, the holes in all levels of defence become aligned the conditions could exist for accidents to occur.

When incidents occur, as with Gina, it is unlikely that that any single action or process was wholly responsible. Reason's model suggests that it is more likely that a series of seemingly minor or even apparently irrelevant events happen, either at the same time or consecutively; the holes align and the combined impact results in a serious and untoward incident. Often people have been working in the same area and environment for long periods of time without event, but the holes existed and the accident was waiting to happen.

(Continued)

(Continued)

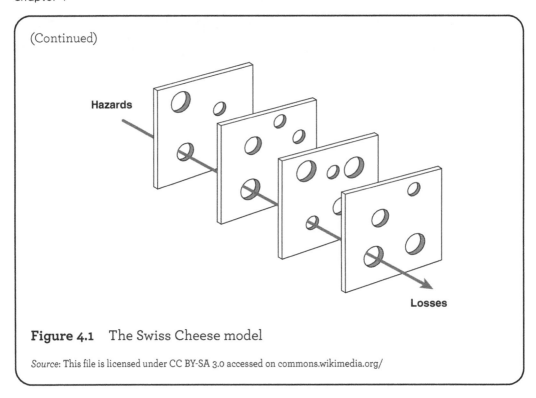

Figure 4.1 The Swiss Cheese model

Source: This file is licensed under CC BY-SA 3.0 accessed on commons.wikimedia.org/

Human factors are not the same as either neglect or incompetence, which is often the perception when things go wrong. The idea of a 'no-blame' culture seeks to recognise that people do not set out to cause accidents or to underperform, and to look for reasons why these things still happen. To address the human and environmental factors that can lead to all the 'holes lining up' is a responsibility of all healthcare professionals; RNAs are no different.

Emotional intelligence and non-technical skills

Even those whose job means that they work alone will, on some level, work and interact with other staff and, obviously, with the patients for whom they care. *Emotional intelligence* is the ability to recognise and manage your own emotions and feelings as well as those of the people around you, and it's built into Platform 1.8 of the Standards.

Psychologist Daniel Goleman (1995) is widely credited with popularising the idea of emotional intelligence; he developed a framework detailing five components that underpin the concept. More importantly, he suggested a range of skills that could be developed, resulting in enhanced emotional intelligence.

The five components are:

1. self-awareness;
2. self-regulation;
3. motivation;
4. empathy;
5. social skills.

Self-awareness

This is an important characteristic in effective leaders – to know and understand your own feelings and emotions means that you can maximise your strengths and be mindful of your shortcomings. Being self-aware enables you to create a fair and inclusive environment, tempers your responses and ensures you ask for help in a timely manner. How you interact with, lead and support people who may have very different ideas and approaches to you is key to safe, effective and harmonious working environments.

Self-regulation

This relates to the capacity to control and direct one's own emotions, to anticipate the consequences of our actions and reduce impulsive responses. This management does not equate to denying or supressing emotions but rather to exercising choice in how those emotions are expressed. Goleman (1998, p. 99) suggests: 'signs of emotional self-regulation ... are not hard to miss: a propensity for reflection and thoughtfulness; comfort with ambiguity; and integrity – an ability to say no to impulsive urges'.

According to White and Grason (2019), self-regulation relates to both what we chose to say to others and how we behave – they describe this as 'behaviour surveillance'. Body language truly is a 'language' and this needs to be considered in interactions with colleagues and with patients and their families. Think about the image of the rushed and harried nurse – head down, bustling past clearly busy and focused but also lacking in engagement and 'saying': 'I am not available and cannot be disturbed.' And, how often have you gone to work feeling perfectly positive and happy to have this feeling dented and even destroyed by the way in which you are greeted by the colleagues that you are taking over from? The language used, the emotions expressed have an enormous impact on those around us and can be regulated.

If you cannot or do not motivate others, then you may struggle to be an effective leader.

Motivation

Everyone can lack motivation at times, but a more pervasive problem has stalked nursing – the idea that nurses 'eat their young' (Meires, 2018; Clark, 2021) and struggle to motivate and elevate their colleagues. Gillespie et al. (2017) made the disheartening claim that this disturbing term has been internationally used and understood by nurses for over 30 years. Motivating yourself and your colleagues is clearly an important and much needed element of an emotionally intelligent leader.

Case study: Zuzanna

Zuzanna is a final year trainee nursing associate (TNA) and started a placement with a community nursing team three weeks previously. There had been several changes in staff in the months preceding this and the team is undergoing a period of settling in and

(Continued)

(Continued)

adapting to the new staff – always an unsettling time. Zuzanna is allocated to various staff members to work alongside, with the overall support of her assessor. However, she becomes increasingly aware that one of the RNAs in the team seems to be avoiding her. Zuzanna feels that the RNA stops talking or leaves abruptly when she enters the room; she also seems to be ignoring her. Zuzanna is in the morning team meeting when her assessor asks the RNA to work with Zuzanna for the day, but the RNA makes an excuse and says she does not have the capacity to support 'the student'. The RNA does not look at Zuzanna, appears to be angry and stressed; when the assessor tries to encourage her to work with Zuzanna, she becomes increasingly angry and, finally, tearfully rushes from the room. Zuzanna is horrified; she feels awkward and embarrassed and as if she is the cause of whatever is troubling the RNA – she doesn't know what to do.

Nurses have always taught and mentored the next generation of their colleagues; it is a common mechanism to provide training that exists across all health professions. However, many students report that the environments they encounter are not always supportive towards students and might not prioritise learning and development for students or for their own staff. Uniquely, students join a team, stay for a short but purposeful period and then leave. This process would challenge the emotional intelligence of the most self-aware and confident person, let alone those who are inexperienced and in training.

Activity 4.5 Communication

The difference between how we see ourselves and others see us

Look again at Figure 3.3 on pp. 55, Johari Window self-awareness framework. Use the Johari Window to list five words that you believe describe who you are as a person. Then ask a friend to also give you five words that they think describe you. Set out the Johari Window and place the words in one of the four categories you think best reflects the description. By doing this you will start to see the similarities but also the difference between how you see yourself and how you are 'seen'!

Perhaps if the RNA in Zuzanna's case had exercised more self-awareness they could have taken a more proactive approach and discussed their needs and concerns earlier? Those staff members who knew the RNA might have recognised behaviours the RNA was not aware of – a perfect opportunity for some compassionate feedback? Either way, and importantly, could the upset and confusion Zuzanna felt have been avoided?

As the exercise is unique to each reader no example has been provided. A link to this idea can be found in the Further reading section.

Empathy

Much has been written in recent years about the importance of empathy (also of compassion, more of that in Chapter 8) and Goleman (1995) identified empathy as an important component of emotional intelligence. Empathy is the ability to recognise and share the thoughts and feelings of another, and this shared understanding is often cited as key to enhancing patient care (McKinnon, 2017) and to working well with colleagues (Hojat et al., 2014). By empathising with patients, their families and with colleagues it is possible to understand their perspective and this understanding can assist in informing how we respond.

Social skills

This relates to the way in which we build relationships with people – the tools we use and qualities we possess that enable us to do this. You may not have appreciated that you have these 'skills', but how you persuade someone, how you initiate or manage change, how you resolve disagreements, communicate unambiguously, collaborate and cooperate and how you inspire and lead colleagues is all down to your social skills.

So, what are these skills? Almost any quality or characteristic that you possess that helps and supports you to form positive, meaningful and productive relationships with others!

Table 4.2 lists these qualities according to Serrat, 2017.

Table 4.2   Social skills

Social skills	
Influence	Individuals with this competence:
	• are skilled at persuasion
	• fine-tune presentations to appeal to the listener
	• use complex strategies like indirect influence to build consensus and support; and
	• orchestrate dramatic events to effectively make a point
Communication	Individuals with this competence:
	• are effective in give-and-take, registering emotional cues in attuning their message
	• deal with difficult issues straightforwardly
	• listen well, seek mutual understanding and welcome sharing of information fully; and
	• foster open communication and stay receptive to bad news as well as good
Leadership	Individuals with this competence:
	• articulate and arouse enthusiasm for a shared vision and mission
	• step forward to lead as needed, regardless of position
	• guide the performance of others while holding them accountable; and
	• lead by example

(Continued)

Table 4.2 (Continued)

Social skills	
Change catalyst	Individuals with this competence:
	• recognise the need for change and remove barriers
	• challenge the status quo to acknowledge the need for change
	• champion the change and enlist others in its pursuit; and
	• model the change expected of others
Conflict management	Individuals with this competence:
	• handle difficult people and tense situations with diplomacy and tact
	• spot potential conflict, bring disagreements into the open and help de-escalate
	• encourage debate and open discussion; and
	• orchestrate win–win solutions
Building bonds	Individuals with this competence:
	• cultivate and maintain extensive informal networks
	• seek out relationships that are mutually beneficial
	• build rapport and keep others in the loop; and
	• make and maintain personal friendships among work associates
Collaboration and cooperation	Individuals with this competence:
	• balance a focus on task with attention to relationships
	• collaborate, sharing plans, information and resources
	• promote a friendly and cooperative climate; and
	• spot and nurture opportunities for collaboration
Team capabilities	Individuals with this competence:
	• model team qualities such as respect, helpfulness and cooperation
	• draw all members into active and enthusiastic participation
	• build team identity, esprit de corps and commitment; and
	• protect the group and its reputation and share credit

Source: Link.springer.com/chapter/10.1007/978-981-10-0983-9_3#chapter-info.

Importantly, social skills and our wider emotional intelligence can also assist us in working with a broad and often varied group of colleagues and patients. The famous Swiss psychoanalyst Carl Jung (1875–1961) said, 'everything that irritates us about others can lead to an understanding of ourselves' (Jung and Jaffe, 1965). All five of the components that underpin the development of our emotional intelligence can help us value diversity, fit in with each other, acknowledge and work with the human strengths and frailties of others. In short – emotional intelligence and our understanding of ourselves helps us respond to the human factors that influence our daily work and our leadership skills.

Cognitive non-technical skills: situational awareness and decision-making

Situational awareness

Very simply, this is your ability to accurately comprehend what is going on in a particular situation or with a particular person or patient. Endsley (1995) described three levels of awareness that build one upon the other:

1. Level 1: perception of elements in the current situation.
2. Level 2: comprehension of the current situation.
3. Level 3: projection of future status.

So, this equates to being aware of all the factors contributing to a situation, working out what is actually happening and then what could happen, depending on how you or others might respond. And this is important because a lack of situational awareness has been highlighted as a barrier to effective management of sick and deteriorating patients (Murray et al., 2019).

Decision-making

The aim of having good situational awareness skills is to benefit appropriate decision-making and, clearly, RNAs need to be able to make safe, accurate and responsive decisions about the care provided to patients. There are several different theories and models to help frame decision-making strategies, but one that is simple and clear relates to the ideas described by Kahneman (2013). Kahneman suggests that there are two types of thinking, that the brain operates using two systems – fast and slow, or System 1 and System 2. Fast, System 1 thinking is described as intuitive, automatic and unconscious and can be seen as a reflex reaction to what is happening around us. This system relies on pattern recognition which relates to previous experience and aligns to the 'gut feeling' of situational awareness. When you are working in routine and expected situations you will be governed by System 1 thinking, which can account for 98 per cent of all our thinking.

Slow, System 2 thinking is much more deliberate and takes conscious effort – it requires you to be rational and analytical. This decision-making will be underpinned by information that is carefully gathered and processed, including both logical interpretation and scepticism as a mechanism for checking and interrogating the available data. Obviously, if System 1 is the mechanism for 98 per cent of our thinking, then System 2 fills the other 2 per cent. On the surface it would seem that System 2 thinking is preferable, more reliable and safer; however, it is, as the name suggests, a slow process and can result in taking too much time to address problems. In fact, Systems 1 and 2 complement each other and both are necessary in daily practice, but System 2 thinking will always override System 1 and will be needed when you are unable to quickly form logical conclusions. The more complex or demanding the situation the more there is an imperative to engage System 2 thinking and decision-making.

And why does it matter? As a leader you need to be aware of what can influence and impact your thinking and decision-making and that of your colleagues. For instance, consider HALT, which stands for Hungry, Angry, Late, Tired (Baverstock and Finlay, 2019) – all very human emotions and situations. If you utilise more System 1 thinking you are more likely to be affected by these situations and your decision-making could be adversely impacted. If you favour System 2 thinking you might be slow to respond to these emotions and you could risk confirmation bias as you may seek to make your deliberations fit your own viewpoint – even if this is illogical.

By being self-aware and by using your social awareness skills you can address these factors – for example, by ensuring that you and your colleagues take breaks, eat regularly and feel comfortable to ask for support. By reflecting on decisions made and asking for confirmation of your conclusions you can assess if you are limiting your findings or being subjective in your reasoning, all of which makes for safer patient care.

Personal non-technical skills: coping with stress and fatigue

In the previous section it was apparent that many factors can have an impact on how we interact with others and how we make decisions. Working in healthcare frequently involves exposure to distressing and challenging situations; staffing and skill-mix pressures increase stressful conditions. The Department of Health devised a strategy, *Compassion in Practice* (Cummings and Bennett, 2012), which contained a raft of actions, the fifth of these aimed to have the 'right staff, with the right skills in the right place' (p. 14). A key factor in achieving this is to ensure effective working patterns and rostering. Twelve-hour shift patterns are widespread throughout the NHS and some research suggests that these can exacerbate fatigue (Ball et al., 2015). According to a recent *NHS Staff Survey* (2021) nearly 40 per cent of NHS staff reported that they struggled to do their jobs properly due to staff shortages and 44 per cent said that they had suffered ill-health due to work-related stress. This is a significant problem and one which has attracted a great deal of discussion and research, especially in terms of patient safety and staff retention and attrition (RCN, 2015; Deakin, 2022).

As an RNA you have two obligations, to address: how you deal with your own stress and any fatigue; and how you acknowledge and support your colleagues who may be experiencing these same pressures (see Proficiency 1.5 in the *Standards of Proficiency* [NMC, 2018c]).

Looking after yourself is not self-indulgent. Professional, modern nursing is just as much a vocation as it ever was, but that does not necessitate neglecting your own needs nor being insensitive to the needs of your colleagues. Nurses are not heroes, they are ordinary people doing an extraordinary job, a job with very real challenges.

Social non-technical skills: communication, team-work and leadership

In 2012 a team of Google employees set out to try and identify what makes a team effective; the initiative was called Project Aristotle after the philosopher's famous quotation that 'the whole is greater than the sum of its parts'. The researchers discovered that what mattered most was less about who is in the team and more about how the team interacts and works together. People needed to feel safe within the team to take risks and to believe that they will not be humiliated or penalised for making mistakes, asking questions, or making suggestions. They also discovered that it was important for teams to take time to chat and to listen to each other – to establish what they termed 'group norms'. When this environment existed, the team was more productive and successful – and this seems so obvious when written down, yet, as you are reading this, you likely agree that this does not always describe the environment in which you work.

Good communication, self-awareness and reflection, role modelling, empathy – in fact, all the elements relevant to human factors and environmental culture described in this chapter – can and will contribute to creating the circumstance where this safety, belief and understanding will exist. As an RNA you have the same level of responsibility and the same capabilities as any other team member to lead and to role model the sort of behaviours that create this environment.

Understanding the theory: situational awareness

Let us apply situational awareness theory to a patient who you are caring for:

- Level 1 means that you notice the individual characteristics or cues in a situation – that is, deteriorating physical observations such as pulse, respiratory rate and conscious level and the resources that you have to hand such as senior colleagues.
- Level 2 means that you can interpret these cues and work out what could be happening – the patient is in heart failure and becoming hypoxic.
- Finally, level 3 results in you using the information you have gathered to work out what happens next – you need to get help to manage this patient, so you alert and inform your senior colleague; the patient needs careful monitoring and so on. Early warning score systems such as the National Early Warning System (NEWS) and surgical safety check lists are essential tools that help support all three levels of situational awareness.

Most errors in situational awareness occur in Level 1 – the failure to accurately perceive the elements of the current situation. This failure is usually due to not having the necessary information and data and this could be for a variety of reasons:

- information that is difficult to gather or find;
- not accessing or obtaining the necessary information;
- information is just not available;
- incomplete information or focusing on one element to the exclusion of wider information;
- misinterpreting or simply not understanding information.

Failures in situational awareness are common and can affect healthcare staff who are novices and who are very experienced. Being an expert means that one is susceptible to confirmation bias as experience can lead to complacency and there is the temptation to see what is expected, to make the facts fit preconceived ideas. Confidence is fine, over-confidence can lead to people not checking or asking for the opinions of others which could result in making the wrong decision. For more novice staff mistakes can happen because they do not know what to look for or, if they do see something, they may not understand what they are seeing or what the implications might be.

While some situational awareness is innate (your 'gut' instincts), there are ways that you, your colleagues and the teams that you work in can maintain and improve this skill. Getting the right information is obviously key and the imperative to do this increases when situations are highly pressured or something unusual happens. Use all the appropriate mechanisms to access and check information and be aware of distractions and interruptions. Ensure that relevant information is transmitted effectively to others and that it is clearly understood.

You also need the ability to check your own understanding; taking a short time out, even – perhaps especially – when busy, to review where you are and what information you have may save significant time later. You need to question your goal and ensure that all those around you are working to the same aim; challenge assumptions and communicate decisions clearly.

Case study: Philip

Philip is an HCA on a busy elderly care ward; he has three children, one of whom has special needs and whose health had been a constant worry since she was born five years ago. The previous week the little girl had undergone surgery to try and correct a heart defect and Philip had taken some compassionate leave from work – today is his first shift back at work following this leave.

When he arrives for work, he finds a card to him and his family from all the ward team has been left in his locker, wishing them well and his daughter a swift recovery. A small soft toy accompanies the card. Several of his colleagues stop to ask how he is and enquire about his daughter, he gets a hug from one and lots of kind and understanding comments from all. The team leader for the shift checks with him quietly and asks how he is feeling; she lets him know he will be working with experienced colleagues that he knows well and that they are adequately staffed for the shift ahead. It is made clear to him that if he struggles in any way, he just needs to ask for help and that he can contact his family any time that he needs to for updates and reassurance. Philip visibly relaxes and reassures everyone that he is fine and happy to be back at work.

The care and consideration shown to Philip seems to indicate the 'group norms' of the ward staff. This approach not only reassures and supports Philip but creates an environment where others, seeing how he is treated, will understand the ward culture and also feel safe and confident. Staff will then, in turn, role model this behaviour, creating the same environment for others and … so it continues.

The environment and how you fit in!

The word *environment* can mean several different things – from the physical structure and layout of a building to the resources and equipment available within a workspace. However, environment also relates to the meaning that people attach to a physical space and the way that they interact with it. In fact, way back in 1997 the RCN developed a programme called Observations of Care to help support their leadership and professional development process. This practice required two observers to use their senses to observe what was happening in a care environment over a given period – highlighting that being in such an environment is a multisensory experience. A person's visual observations will be augmented by what they smell, hear and feel, and all these elements will create a relationship with the environment.

As an RNA you will be able to influence the physical environment – you may be involved in audits relating to staffing or patient safety. All equipment used in nursing is required to meet specific safety standards and you may be required to undertake assessments of equipment or liaise with medical electronics or maintenance colleagues to ensure continued safe standards. You will need to be aware of the standards for all the equipment you use and when and how often maintenance and updates are required.

Understanding the theory: PUWER and LOLER

There are a number of laws and guidelines that relate to the safety of the physical environment in which you work. PUWER is an abbreviation of the Provision and Use of Work Equipment Regulations 1998. The PUWER regulation aims to ensure the safety of people as well as companies operating, maintaining and having control over equipment and machinery used in their workplaces. Equipment such as infusion pumps, air filtration systems, patient monitoring machines, photocopiers and personal protective equipment – in fact, any equipment you use to carry out your work – is

(Continued)

(Continued)

likely to fall under PUWER regulations. LOLER stands for Lifting Operating and Lifting Equipment Regulations 1998 – and specifically relate to lifting equipment; it includes a requirement for regular training and is why you carry out yearly, mandatory manual handling training.

While the physical environment is clearly important it is also essential that the culture of the working environment be considered. Hopefully, this chapter has highlighted how impactful that culture can be for those who work within it and, crucially, for those who are cared for by these people. Whether there is a psychologically and emotionally safe environment to work in, whether there is a learning culture, whether the team work well together, whether non-technical skills are valued as much as technical skills – all these aspects will impact on the environment and this, in turn, will influence patient care. The tone and culture of an environment can be set and influenced by the leadership provided to and by the team – all RNAs can impact this culture by contributing their experience and skill to lead colleagues and care.

Chapter summary

This chapter has provided you with an introduction to the concepts of human and environmental factors, with definitions and examples. As an RNA you may work in any number of different areas and specialities, yet the skills required to address the challenges of working with your fellow human beings in all environments and cultures will be similar. You have been provided with information and examples that human factors relate to the nature of your job, to you as an individual and to the organisation you work for and that when circumstances align failures in any one of these areas can result in significant harm. Resources and activities should enable you to explore these ideas further and to take the opportunity to evaluate your own non-technical skills – cognitive, personal and social – to assist you with situational awareness and decision-making. Finally, this chapter should encourage you to understand that the environment you work in is more than simply your physical surroundings and that you as a leader can impact the culture and outcomes of your workplace.

Activities: brief outline answers

Activity 4.1

Human factors:

- tired due to disturbed sleep;
- rushing;

- impacted by the distress of the bereaved relative;
- forgetting to sign for medication dispensed;
- RN assuming rather than checking.

Environmental factors:

- colleague is newly qualified, therefore lacks experience;
- several patients with high levels of acuity;
- bells ringing;
- patient who did not question being given two lots of medication.

Relevant NMC Standards: 1.1, 1.2, 1.3, 1.12

This is not an exhaustive list as many Standards have elements that are relevant to this scenario – however, these are the most significant and broadly relevant.

Activity 4.2

Example and non-exhaustive answer based on a relatively newly qualified RNA working in an emergency department:

Table 4.3 Answers to the job, the individual, the organisation

The job	The individual	The organisation
Unpredictable due to nature of emergency admissions	Some admissions can be very distressing and this causes upset	Significant number of staffing vacancies
Often highly demanding patient group	Level of confidence	Policy of no corridor nursing, therefore patients kept in ambulances for long periods
Can be very unwell or seriously injured patients	Lack of pattern recognition – a lot of patients have conditions/ injuries not seen by the RNA before	Change in shift pattern that has caused issues with childcare for relevant staff
Some patients cannot provide information as unconscious or have cognitive issues	Hard to delegate to others due to perceived junior status and lack of experience	Lack of understanding of the RNA role from colleagues
Having the right person in the right place – not all staff can be skilled in all aspects of emergency care	Tries to prove capabilities but does not always ask for help as feels it will confirm lack of experience	

Activity 4.3

1. Risk to the patient; first, risk of infection as clearly infection control policies were not being followed. Other risks to patient safety include: lack of easily accessible information, staff who feel disengaged or unsure of what they need to do, a nurse-in-charge who is distracted and not present on the ward. This can obviously lead to mistakes in all aspects of a patient's care – misidentification, drug errors, delays in treatment – the list is almost endless.

2. Human factors:

   - level of experience of the staff on duty;
   - distraction – trying to contact others to support the shift;
   - unfamiliarity with colleagues – a team that is not used to working together;
   - clinical practice – not adhering to infection control procedures;
   - poor communication.

   Environmental factors:

   - staff without adequate training and induction;
   - skill mix;
   - staff shortage;
   - lack of clarity relating to ward procedures and equipment;
   - access to patent information.

3. Relevant NMC Standards: 1.1, 1.2, 1.3, 2.9

Again, this is not an exhaustive list as many Standards have elements that are relevant to this scenario; however, these are the most significant and broadly relevant.

Activity 4.4

Failures in specifically *non-technical skills* re. Gina's story.
   The factors which led to the error include:

- *complacency* – the process had been the same for a long time and there had been no reviews or consideration of human or environmental factors;
- *distraction/situational awareness* – the catheter fell to the floor distracting staff who then drew up the wrong solution;
- *failure to check* – the doctor assumed the solution they had received was what they had asked for and did not check;
- *situational awareness* – after the first signs that something was wrong occurred no root cause was discovered and so the mistake was repeated;
- *the procedure was carried out correctly from a technical perspective* – the mistakes which led to such pain and suffering for the patient were entirely human and environmental. See the relevant video in the Useful websites section for further discussion about what caused this error.

Further reading

What Google Learned from its Quest to Build the Perfect Team: **www.nytimes. com/2016/02/28/magazine/what-google-learned-from-its-quest-to-build-the-perfect-team.html**

This is a link to an article about why and how Project Aristotle got underway. There are some interesting stories about the real people involved in the study and their experiences.

N.B. *New York Times* is usually a pay-per-view website but you can access this article at least once for free before any request for payment!

Patient Safety First (2010) *Implementing Human Factors in Healthcare*. Available at: Human-Factors-How-to-Guide-v1.2 (3) (1).pdf

This is an easy-to-understand guide to how to implement human factors principles, including some very relevant examples that link to nursing practice.

RCN (2015) The case for Healthy Workplaces: Healthy Workplace, Healthy You. London: RCN. **www.rcn.org.uk/Professional-Development/publications/pub-004963**

RCN document on creating healthy workplaces; some useful links to environmental factors.

Useful websites

https://chfg.org/the-human-factor-learning-from-ginas-story/

This link opens a video of a head of Risk and Safety leading a presentation about what was learned from Gina's story.

www.communicationtheory.org/the-johari-window-model/

This link opens an interesting website which explains how to use the Johari Window.

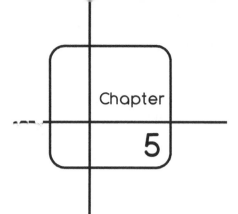

Chapter

5

Understanding data and information for effective care and leadership

Natalie Cusack

Chapter aims

After reading this chapter you will be able to:

• identify current digital health agenda in healthcare and what digital literacy means to the role of a nursing associate (NA);

- understand the legal, ethical and professional issues that relate to healthcare data and information;
- use and recommend evidence-based healthcare resources and share information;
- consider ethics, risk and your role in leadership for a digitally literate workforce.

Introduction

We live in an ever-changing digital society. From the way we shop, bank, watch media and book holidays, digital technology has changed how we access services and organise our lives. The need for Digital First healthcare has been recognised since the summary of the *Five Year Forward View* (NHS England, 2017). Digital technology has potential to open new possibilities, improving the prevention, care and treatment of disease, and refining service delivery across healthcare (NHS England, 2019).

In the nursing profession, the gathering, processing and sharing of data and information is not a new concept. Documentation of nurse–patient interactions in patient records has given voice to the importance of nursing interventions in patient safety and recovery from disease (Warren, 2013, p. 171). Advancements in health information technology have been changing the way we manage, communicate and access health data and information, prompting a requirement for nursing competency in digital information literacy (Staggers et al., 2002; RCN, 2018; Brown et al., 2020).

In order to 'practise effectively', the NMC *Code* (2018a) requires us to:

- practise in line with the best available evidence;
- communicate clearly;
- work cooperatively;
- share your skills, knowledge and experience for the benefit of people receiving care and your colleagues;
- keep clear and accurate records relevant to your practise.

The aim of this chapter is to explore how to practise in accordance with the NMC *Code* (2018a) within a digital world. You will be introduced to current healthcare agenda and key legislation that protects personal information. While record keeping is an important skill for healthcare professionals, the ability to navigate the abundance of health information for evidence-based resources is imperative in our role as a patient advocate. Furthermore, a rapidly changing digital world requires NAs to develop their own digital literacy and leadership skills. As the RCN (2018) says, every nurse is an e-nurse.

Digital agenda in healthcare and nursing

To appreciate the role of data and information in our workplace it might be helpful to explore current initiatives in healthcare and nursing practice across the United Kingdom.

The NHS *Five Year Forward View* (NHS England, 2017) set out recommendations for a sustainable service that is adapted to the challenges of modern healthcare. The report covers a wide set of recommendations from the integration of health and social care services to improved pathways for emergency care. Throughout the review, the theme of utilising new technology is frequent and proposes advances to the integration of services, delivery of health promotion and enabling patients' greater control of their care.

Harnessing new technology means using computers, software and applications available to enhance your ability to deliver good-quality care to patients. As a TNA, you will recognise that providing effective person-centred care requires us to consider our personal skills, care environment and care process for good person-centred outcomes (McCance and McCormack, 2016).

Advancements in technology have changed the way we collect, understand and disseminate information. An example which you may be familiar with is the introduction of electronic health records used to document the clinical information of patients receiving care. Clear and accurate recording and sharing information has long been recognised in the NMC *Code* (2018a) to preserve the safety of those in our care. Since the increase in the use of electronic health records across the NHS, there have been advantages and barriers to its use for clinicians; we will discuss some of these later in this chapter.

The summary of the *Five Year Forward View* (NHS England, 2017) reiterates the benefits of effectively using new digital technologies including smartphone apps, software such as records systems, online tools and wearable medical devices (NICE, 2018). The use of digital technology ranges from the management of long-term conditions to empowering the public to access evidence-based health information. Digital health technology should not replace nursing skill, but it should augment our practice and reduce inefficiency, supporting organisation of clinician time, and reducing waste. Another recognised benefit of digital health technology is the gathering, organisation and accessibility of data that informs decisions for service improvement and future health research. Collection of data should inform your decisions when reviewing quality of care and implementing ways to improve services, in line with the *Healthcare Leadership Model* (NHS Leadership Academy, 2013), as will be discussed later in this chapter.

Following the *Five Year Forward View* (NHS England, 2017), *The NHS Long Term Plan* (NHS England, 2019) proposed that the NHS should be a Digital First organisation, offering digital solutions for people accessing services and those who work across the NHS. The plan continues recommendations made in its predecessor and sets out expectations that NHS services be 'digital ready' by 2024. *The NHS Long Term Plan* (NHS England, 2019) highlights that digital transformation must achieve the following:

- *Empowering the public*

The use of digital technology enables the public to take greater control over their health and well-being. This might look like booking GP appointments online, ordering repeat prescriptions or monitoring long-term health conditions through mobile applications.

- *Supporting health and care professionals*

Digital technology should be easy to use and reliable. Staff should have access to training and opportunities to give feedback on the technology they use.

- *Supporting clinical care*

Digital technology should provide seamless support both to clinicians and service users; it should enhance our practice, improving efficiency and giving us more time to care for patients.

- *Improving public health*

The potential to gather large amounts of data across the health service will provide valuable information for future research. When you are updating care plans, completing assessments and conducting an audit, the information you have collected provides an evidence-based contribution to the commissioning of new services, or understanding the epidemiology of disease.

- *Improving clinical safety and efficiency*

Finally, digital technology should make healthcare safer for everyone. Using new technology should enable clinicians to access, communicate and share patient information in real time. Technology has the potential to reduce error and recognise the warning signs of patient deterioration.

Activity 5.1   Reflection

Go to the *NHS Long Term Plan* (NHS England, 2019) and read Chapter 5, 'Digitally-enabled care will go mainstream across the NHS'.

Take ten minutes to make a list of the digital technology you have seen on your practice placements or workplace.

What purpose do these tools have according to the highlights of the digital transformation plan?

You can find the *NHS Long Term Plan* (NHS England, 2019) in the Further reading section at the end of this chapter.

As this activity is based on your own observation, there is no outline answer at the end of the chapter.

Covid-19 and digital transformation

In 2020 the Covid-19 pandemic rapidly changed how healthcare is delivered and pushed digital healthcare into the public agenda. The use of telemedicine, virtual consultations and remote monitoring of patients became common in the way we access and deliver healthcare (Peek et al., 2020). Some of the changes are potentially irreversible, prompting the need for nursing professionals to adapt their use of digital skills (Barrett and Heale, 2021). The Covid-19 pandemic also highlighted how accessible public health information and the spread of 'misinformation' impacts disease outcomes and the nursing profession

(Mitchell, 2021). As a nursing associate, enabling your patients to access evidence-based information and advocating for those who face digital inequality will be a prominent challenge across your career.

In 2019 the *Topol Review* was published by Health Education England (HEE, 2019a); the paper predicts three major changes to how healthcare will be delivered by 2040. The technology that will impact healthcare's future is predicted to be telemedicine, artificial intelligence (AI) and genomic sequencing. This future-facing document has big plans for healthcare, but, while we are not quite at the stage where AI can support complex clinical decision-making, for these innovations to take place, good-quality data and a digitally literate workforce is essential. If you are interested in finding out more about future prediction for technologies role in health, *The Topol Review* (HEE, 2019a) is listed in the further reading section.

The RCN (2018) recognises that innovation starts with enabling the current and future workforce to develop confidence and capability in their own digital literacy skills, transforming the nurse profession from using technology as a process we do, to knowing and creating solutions to clinical problems with the help of digital technology. For the nursing profession to take these steps and manage its own innovation, a foundation must be in place to promote trust and confidence in the systems we use.

Understanding the theory: the *Digital Capabilities Framework* (2017)

In 2017, HEE launched its *Digital Capabilities Framework* as a guide for healthcare employers and professionals to measure their digital literacy skills and identify areas for improvement. The framework has five domains which encompass digital literacy in the aspect of safety, security, well-being and identity. You can access the framework in the further reading section.

Ask yourself: how do you feel your digital literacy skills match up to the framework?

- *Information, data and media literacies*: This domain relates to your ability to find, manage, store and share digital information. As an NA you are trusted with the collection, storage and processing of personal and private data; at times this personal information needs to be shared for cohesive care. You should develop understanding on how this can be done safely.
- *Teaching, learning and self-development*: Can you use digital tools for professional and personal development? This could be as simple as completing your information governance training online or attending a global conference in the comfort of your own home. If you are tech savvy, are you able to support your co-workers to improve their digital skills?
- *Communication, collaboration and participation*: The communication domain relates to your ability to use and effectively communicate with digital tools. Are you able to use email, forums and social media safely? Can you maintain your professionalism in a digital environment?
- *Technical proficiency*: This domain relates to your competency with tech such as computers, phones and software. Your technical proficiency relates to how quickly

you can adapt to new devices and software. When you get a new phone, can you intuitively explore all its features based on previous mobile technology you have used. These skills are transferable to the digital health technology you will encounter over your career.

- *Creation, innovation and scholarship*: It is recognised that a new generation of workforce and student health professionals will bring new skills to the profession (Wong et al., 2021). Everyone in the nursing profession should be encouraged to create solutions to clinical problems they encounter and comment on technology they use.

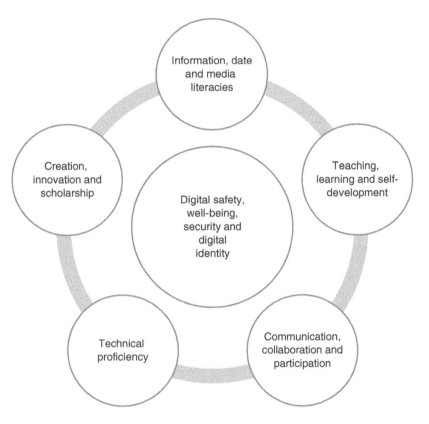

Figure 5.1   Digital Capabilities Framework

Source: Adapted from Beetham (2017).

Activity 5.2   Reflection

Digital literacy will become increasingly important to your career. As a TNA, you will have the opportunity to develop your digital skills through study, assignments and online learning platforms utilised by your higher education institution. Adapting to

(Continued)

(Continued)

digital platforms during training will enable you to develop study skills that will directly benefit your journey to become an RNA.

Using the *Digital Capabilities Framework* (HEE, 2017), consider the skills you have developed over the duration of your programme; where could you improve in the future?

As this activity is based on your own observation, there is no outline answer at the end of the chapter.

What is patient data and information and why is it important?

So, what does data and information have to do with you in your role as TNA and leader? We are not quite at the stage where AI is supporting us to make complex clinical decisions; however, this technology does rely on good-quality clinical data that the nursing profession deals with in their daily role.

Data is raw facts, unorganised numbers, statistics, values, or symbols gathered which separately may not make sense. Data we gather must be organised to build information which has a meaning for us. Let's put this into a healthcare context with the case study below.

Case study: Imani

Imani is a TNA working in a medical assessment unit, overseeing a six-bedded bay. Admitted to her bay is 67-year-old Andrea, after a suspected myocardial infarction; Andrea requires close monitoring.

Imani has been asked to record Andrea's physical observations.

As a single number, the pulse rate Imani has recorded might not tell her much about Andrea's condition; however, when Imani has the rest of the vital signs, clinically significant information becomes clear to her. She records those physical observations every four hours over a 24-hour period. The observation measure is the data; once collected, stored and processed, Imani has information on Andrea's condition. The more data she collects, the clearer the information on Andrea's condition will be.

Imani continues to work with Andrea over the next three days; during this time she is continuously recording health data that will enable the clinical team to provide safe, effective and person-centred care.

Activity 5.3   Reflection

What other data might Imani collect to monitor Andrea's condition?

Suggested answers will be provided at the end of this chapter.

The process of recording and storing data builds patient information, which is stored as health records. The Data Protection Act (2018) defines a *health record* as a record which consists of data concerning health and has been made by, or on behalf of, a health professional in connection with the diagnosis, care or treatment of the individual to whom the data relates. The medium in which this information is recorded will inevitably vary between NHS trusts and private providers. However, the legal and professional issues we need to explore will be applicable to health and care providers across the United Kingdom.

Electronic health records

If you have previous experience as a healthcare support worker, you may have used paper records in the past, or even a mix of paper and electronic ones. Electronic health records (EHRs) are prominently used across healthcare settings; as previously mentioned, a target for the *NHS Long Term Plan* (NHS England, 2019) is for all NHS services to be using EHRs by 2024.

As an NA, you must be competently trained and fully aware of your personal responsibility in maintaining and managing health records (NHS, 2021); training should be provided by your employer. The benefits of EHRs are their ability to protect data in accordance with legislation, which will be covered later in this chapter. Information can be accessible in real time to clinicians who need it and, increasingly, service users get access to their medical records through mobile applications such as the NHS app. The success of a new technology depends on its perceived usefulness, trust and ease of use (Pavlou, 2003). Across the United Kingdom, clinicians have reported that their EHRs are difficult to use, duplicate work and can crash or update at inappropriate times, obviously causing annoyance to everyone involved!

Activity 5.4   Critical thinking

As both a trainee and RNA, you are expected to provide leadership and role modelling to junior staff, which you will read about further in Chapter 8. Consider the following scenario.

It is Monday morning and you have returned after a long weekend off; you are delegated your usual bay of six patients in the Medical Assessment Unit. This morning

(Continued)

(Continued)

you have been asked to prepare for the Multidisciplinary Team (MDT) board round at 10am. You need to prepare for the doctor and update yourself with patient progress over the weekend.

Toni was the Support Worker in your bay last night; she has completed her end of shift notes for her patient John, a 76-year-old gentleman admitted on Friday.

Sunday Nocte Shift

John was settled overnight. He was assisted to wash and dress in the evening as per care plan, but John was difficult and resistive to the assistance.

His sleep was broken as John expressed discomfort, all physical observation in normal range.

John is asleep at time of note.

What information do you feel is missing from this entry and does it help your board round preparation?

Reflect on how you could approach Toni to support her.

Suggested answers are available at the end of this chapter.

Legal, ethical and professional issues that relate to healthcare data and information

As part of your role and registration, you have privileged access to personal information, including medical history, family contacts, MDT consultations, care plans and general conversation about fluctuating feelings throughout the day. Furthermore, the NMC proficiencies for NAs (2018c) require clear and accurate records are made and shared appropriately across the MDT. It is important to recognise that we have a legal obligation to safeguard the sensitive data and information we manage. You will receive regular mandatory 'information governance' training in your workplace, but it is important to cover the basics of data protection in this chapter.

As will be discussed in Chapter 6, you are accountable not only for your own practice but also your delegation and leadership responsibilities. This will mean that data breaches can result in penalties on your registration, or even a financial penalty! So, let's cover three key topics of data and the law.

Data protection

Personal data is a collection of information about an individual who is identifiable through factors such as name, location and other identification methods (e.g., NHS number). This information usually relates the person's physical, psychological and social identity (Data Protection Act, 2018). Not all data is equal, there are stronger protections for sensitive information, such as race, ethnic background, political opinion, religious beliefs, biometrics and health; information that we consider part of our holistic nursing assessment.

Due to rapidly changing technologies designed to store data and share information, new legislation determines the responsibility of organisations, such as the NHS and the individuals who work there, yourself. As an NA, you need to be aware of current legislation and the impact to your role and the rights of those under your duty of care.

The two key documents you should be aware of are the Data Protection Act (2018) which is the current law in the United Kingdom regarding personal information. The UK General Data Protection Regulation (UK GDPR, 2018) instructs organisations on how to manage personal data within the law. The basic principles that you need to be aware of for data protection in your workplace are that data should be:

- used fairly, lawfully and transparently;
- used for a specified, explicit purpose;
- used in a way that is adequate, relevant and limited to only what is necessary;
- accurate and, where necessary, kept up to date and kept for no longer than is necessary;
- handled in a way that ensures appropriate security, including protection against unlawful or unauthorised processing, access, loss, destruction or damage.

(Spencer and Patel, 2019)

These principles of GDPR should be considered while you are collecting, managing and sharing data between your team members and if required, a wider multiagency team. Which brings us onto our second consideration of lawful data protection.

Access and information sharing

To promote effective care, you will need to share patient information with those who need it as per Platform 1.11 of Annexe A of the NMC Standards (2018c): 'provide clear verbal, digital or written information and instructions when sharing information, delegating, or handing over responsibility for care'.

The guiding principles for confidentiality and sharing patient information are outlined by *The Caldicott Principles* (National Data Guardian, 2020). While these principles are not a legal requirement, they do support lawful data protection. When sharing personal information, you need to think critically on the purpose of sharing the information, ensuring what you are sharing is necessary and justified.

Patient rights of access to their healthcare information

The GDPR and Data Protection Act allow patients to request to see their medical records. This does not mean they have the right to request you to let them scroll through their digital notes; a request should be made in writing and be approved by the team responsible for the secure management of records (Sullivan and Garland, 2013).

Each trust will have a policy to support patients to access their health records; it may be worth checking your workplace policy for future reference.

With the increase in use of EHRs, some systems do allow for patients to have access to their records without making a formal request. The NHS app enables patients to access their GP records; however, this service does vary between GP surgeries. Under the Freedom of Information Act (2000) patients and staff can request access to any correspondence about them. This includes emails, letters, hand-over notes and text messages. For this reason, it is important to always remain professional and ensure all records are accurate and non-judgemental. When entering a digital note, consider the language you are using and remain objective. Recent research shows that patient accessible health records could positively impact on patient satisfaction, engagement and safety, but ongoing studies are recommended (Neves, et al., 2020).

Activity 5.5   Reflection

Consider the following scenario.

You hear that a famous singer has been spotted in the accident and emergency department; your colleague saw him when she came back from her break. Excited, your team start looking on the EHR to find more information on his visit.

Do you think the relevant legislation and guidance have been followed?

What would be your action be as an RNA?

You can find the answer at the end of this chapter.

Collecting data for service improvement and clinical audit

Throughout this book, you have been introduced to qualities of leadership; if you think back to the Healthcare Leadership model (NHS Leadership Academy, 2013) introduced in Chapter 2, *harnessing information* is introduced to prompt leaders to 'think in an informed way about how to develop proposals for improvement'.

During your studies to become an RNA, you should have the opportunity to participate in the collection of data for clinical audit (NMC, 2018a). Clinical audit is an essential role of the healthcare professional and can be undertaken by any member of the MDT. As part of your leadership role, you may decide to monitor the quality of your service by organising a clinical audit. The process for audit, NICE Quality Standards and the NHS Outcomes Framework will be covered in detail in Chapter 7.

Quality data has the potential to improve services and the data you collect while delivering patient care contributes to enhancing safety, ensuring standards and longevity of your service through commissioning. You are contributing towards clinical audit in every record you make. For this reason, you should ensure that you and your team's clinical records are accurate, complete, relevant, reliable, timely and valid (Dixon and Pearce, 2011).

Data collection for clinical audit can be collected in retrospect where it already exists, and you have access to it – for example, in clinical notes. You also have the option to collect prospective data, a process where data is collected moving forwards (Chambers and Wakley, 2005).

An example of a Quality Standard you may be familiar with is reducing the formation of pressure ulcers – a clinical incentive across primary, secondary and social care. The following case study will demonstrate why data is important to clinical audit.

Activity 5.6   In practice

At the beginning of the chapter, you were asked to consider the care of Andrea who was admitted to the ward with a suspected myocardial infarction. On her admission Andrea is required to be assessed for her risk of developing a hospital-acquired pressure ulcer, in concordance with the NICE guidelines (2015).

You are delegated to complete the admission paperwork, including a pressure ulcer risk assessment.

How would you achieve this, maintaining standards set by the NICE guidelines.

What is the importance of completing the assessment and documentation from a data and information perspective?

You will find the answers at the end of this chapter.

This was a brief introduction to the use of quality data in service improvement, aimed to give you an understanding of the importance of your documentation and record keeping. We will revisit these topics in Chapter 7.

Accessing and communicating information in digital landscapes

At the beginning of the chapter, you were introduced to the *Digital Capabilities Framework* (HEE, 2017); after reading this far, you should have developed insight into the importance of data to your role as a NA. The next step we need to consider is how we use information. This section will cover two topics: sharing sensitive patient information with those who need it and the contemporary issue of accessing quality information, avoiding misinformation and empowering your patients to navigate health information in the virtual environment.

You should already have a good idea about sharing patient information with your colleagues and wider MDT. Your organisation will give you access to a secure email account for the purpose of your role, and IT equipment will be installed with encryption software to keep sensitive information safe. It is essential that you only use your organisational email to send and receive sensitive information.

Case study: phishing

It's 07:00am and Jess checks her mobile phone over her morning coffee. She has an email from an email address she does not recognise. The email claims to be from an old family friend who has reached out to tell Jess a huge fortune awaits. All Jess needs to do is pay a bank holder fee to release the money and a significant percentage of the trapped fortune is hers! She laughs and deletes the email; this is a well-known scam and she's not going to fall for it.

Later that day, Jess checks her emails at work. There is a new email from an address claiming to be the finance team in the hospital, although the email address does not match her employer. They email her 'Urgent, unpaid invoice. I need authorization for this order. Please open the following link to provide a signature'. This looks official, but she feels uneasy. 'Why would they be contacting me over an unpaid invoice, who is this person, I have not spoken to this team before?'

Scams are becoming sophisticated and lure you into opening links or responding to password requests. If you are unsure about a request for your passwords or link, consider checking with your IT department.

Phishing is a cyber security attack where users are tricked into accessing malicious software, links or websites. These attacks can install ransomware, sabotage systems and steal confidential information (National Cyber Security Centre, 2022). Your organisation should have its own policy to protect itself from a cyber-attack and you should receive information on how to protect yourself and how to report suspicious emails.

In 2017 the NHS experienced its largest cyber-attack, the WannaCry ransomware attack, which affected 60 NHS trusts across England and Scotland causing significant disruption and delays (Triggle, 2017). The attack spread through a flaw in Microsoft software and spread automatically (National Audit Office, 2018) rather than through staff email; however, the damage it caused highlights the importance of cyber security in healthcare.

The people who use health services are vulnerable to phishing scams, particularly in the current economic environment post-Covid-19 and the cost of living crisis. NHS Digital (2021a) warn of increasing scams via text message which can impact vulnerable individuals. As a TNA, you should be vigilant to scams to be able to advise and support people under your care. In our personal and professional lives, we are using increasing digital technology to communicate with each other, from social media to applications. As a leader in healthcare, you need to start thinking about your methods of communication with other professionals and people in your care.

Let's consider a scenario: you are working in a community mental health team and have been allocated a new service user to your caseload, 22-year-old Karim. Karim asks you if you use WhatsApp, as this is the best way to keep in contact with him. What professional, legal and security issues may we need to consider while negotiating a communication method with Karim?

Your communication predicament begins with protecting your personal information and maintaining professional boundaries. If you have not been given a suitable phone with access to WhatsApp, you shouldn't be giving Karim your personal number in any circumstance. The NMC (2022, p. 3) provides guidance to its registrants on avoiding unprofessional behaviour on social media, including 'building or pursuing relationships with patients or service users'. If you use your own contact details or social media accounts to communicate with service uses and their families, you are potentially making yourself vulnerable to complaint and blurring the boundaries of your role.

Let's say you have a smartphone device to use for your role; what applications can you use? The NMC (2022) recognises that in some circumstances off the shelf applications, such as WhatsApp, may be a useful tool to engage with service users. Karim is a good example; he may otherwise be hard to engage with, and you want to adapt to his personal needs and preferences. Under these circumstances it is advisable to risk assess and carefully plan your communication decisions and seek advice from your local information governance team (NMC, 2022). WhatsApp (2022) messages are encrypted, and the content cannot be seen by third parties (including WhatsApp) so there is some privacy between content shared. As a TNA, you are not expected to know the full details of confidentiality and privacy of social media and application, but it is wise to work within NMC (2022) guidance and seek support from your information governance office when needed.

Accessing evidence-based information

Access to social media and online health information has created an information wall for health professionals and the public. From bloggers and self-diagnosis tools to non-profit health information websites, the public can be faced with an overwhelming choice of information while seeking advice on their health and well-being. As a clinician, you may want to provide some health promotion and advise resources for your patients to use in their own time. As a leader, you need to demonstrate critical analysis to the resources that you use and potentially recommend, asking the questions of its safety, security and validity. If a patient approaches you about health information received through social media platforms, such as TikTok, what approach would you take?

Improving health literacy in adults is known to reduce health inequality and improve a person's ability to manage their long-term conditions (National Institute of Health Research, 2022). To combat health literacy and provide public access to quality evidence-based information, the NHS launched its NHS Choices website in 2007 with the NHS app launched in 2018. The website and app are designed for the public to access health information, seek advice, book appointments and access their own health records. In 2021 the application's use in the United Kingdom was growing (NHS Digital, 2021b); however, online and mobile health (mHealth) usability and potential to create further health inequality has been questioned.

Activity 5.7 Research

The rise of mHealth has the potential to improve health literacy, deliver public health messages and manage long-term conditions. You may be using mobile applications and online resources to support your own health and well-being – an application for calorie counting, sleep tracking, or step counting. Consider the applications and online resources you use and make a list.

Ask yourself: are these evidence-based interventions?

Would I recommend these to individuals receiving healthcare?

If you have institutional access to journals through Athens or Shibboleth you might search for mHealth applications in a topic of interest, such as 'mHealth' and 'diabetes', or 'mHealth' and 'smoking cessation'; the wealth of literature testing feasibility, usability and validity of mHealth application is rapidly growing.

As this activity is based on your own observation, there is no outline answer at the end of the chapter.

For patient information, use of the NHS resources is usually enough. However, if you want to access evidence-based information for your own knowledge and development, you will want to use a resource for clinicians and healthcare professionals. The NICE website provides a useful source of information, best guidance, research papers and quality standards that we should be using wherever we practise.

You might want to reflect on the recent Covid-19 pandemic as it holds valuable examples of the challenge in disseminating the best available evidence rapidly, as well as the power of misinformation. The Covid-19 pandemic led to an increase in health research thrust into the public eye, leading to speculation, confusion and mistrust over changing advice and conflicting claims (The Lancet Rheumatology, 2021). While misinformation is not new (Russell, 2021), the prevalence of misinformation in the pandemic endangered lives and caused mistrust in healthcare services and professionals. Notable risks were medication shortages due to misinformation, leading to people with the long-term condition rheumatoid arthritis being without their medication and, in the United Kingdom, members of the public filmed inside hospitals, breaking confidentiality and standards of dignity for those accessing services.

Despite the challenges of misinformation and questionable health sources, the public ability to question the status quo could be seen as positive, encouraging more people to actively take interest in their health and treatment options. Russell (2021) advises that misinformation should be combated with compassion, listening and understanding. As a TNA, you may work with patients who present you with health information that is incorrect. It is vital to explore with them the reason it may be untrustworthy and advise reliable resources to access, including NHS Choices or the public section of Cochrane library.

Ethics, risks and leadership in a digital landscape

Over the past decade the expansion of digital technology has developed the way we practise faster than regulation and ethics can keep up with. As with any novel science, there will be risk among the benefits. Registered nurses and NAs have a place in actively reviewing risks, advocating for patients and leading with changes. A recent review from the Queen's Nursing Institute (2022) identifies significant barriers in the adoption of digital health technology: aspects such as poor resources, low connectivity and reducing patient care to 'task-based nursing' where schedules dictate diaries, and premade care plans reduce interactions to tick box exercises. You may have your own examples of how digital technology has negatively impacted your role and patient care.

The Topol Review (HEE, 2019a) also highlighted ethical complications of a digital future. Technology has the potential to make clinical decisions, diagnose and instruct care. Without consideration an *automation bias* could occur where health professionals rely heavily on automated systems, such as computer algorithms or decision support tools, without questioning their recommendations or outputs. This can occur when healthcare professionals trust that the system is reliable and accurate, which may lead them to overlook or dismiss contradictory information or data (Lyell et al., 2017).

Data protection, security and trust has been covered in depth throughout the chapter; however, moving into the future with data powering AI and health research, health service users must be informed, consent to and trust those who hold their data. Digital technology needs data to advance and create algorithms, but AI can only be as knowledgeable as the data entered, leading to a risk of bias and discrimination. People of minority ethnic groups may be disadvantaged by AI and a digital technology could be culturally inappropriate (Wiens et al., 2019).

Across your career you will begin to see changes in the way healthcare is practised. You may be introduced to new initiatives developed to support patient care or gather information for the purpose of audit. As a registrant and leader, you will find yourself managing change, critically evaluating the tools provided and supporting your colleagues who are not confident in their digital capability. Importantly, you must be mindful of preserving disadvantaged voices and maintaining compassionate and empathetic care in your practice.

Digital inequalities exist for both staff and patient populations. For patient groups, digital inequality can impact those already at risk of health inequality, such as people in lower socio-economic groups or who speak English as a second language. Patient groups recommend that health services offer intervention to vulnerable communities to empower digital literacy skills and offer choice (Patient Coalition for AI, Data and Digital Tech in Health, 2022). As an NA, you may be able to advise or lead on a digital skills workshop in your practice area; it may be a discussion to have with your digital transformation lead. Generally, research highlights that patient groups want to develop their digital skills (Betts et al., 2019); projects such as digital cafés are successful at engaging communities.

You can consider taking on additional roles to support the delivery and innovation of digital healthcare within your practice. Digital champions are individuals who are passionate about the use of technology and its potential to improve healthcare services. They encourage others to become more involved in the use of technology in healthcare and help to promote and support digital initiatives within the NHS. Digital champions play a key role in driving innovation and adoption of digital solutions in healthcare, helping to ensure that technology is used effectively to improve patient care and support healthcare professionals in their work.

The NHS Digital Academy, which is part of Health Education England, offers a Digital Champions Programme aimed at developing the digital skills and knowledge of healthcare professionals, encouraging their participation and interest in digital healthcare. The programme aims to build a community of digital champions who can support the implementation of digital healthcare solutions in their organisations and help to drive transformational change in healthcare.

Becoming a digital champion would give an opportunity to develop leadership and management skills, career development and access to an innovative and exciting area of healthcare. The NHS Digital Academy is listed in the further reading section.

Chapter summary

Over this chapter, we have explored what data, information and digital literacy skills mean for your role and your future as an RNA. Clear, accurate and timely data and information plays an essential part in keeping patient safe, providing effective care and transforming our services.

You have a responsibility to protect public personal information, keep records legally and communicate information where deemed necessary. You should advise your patients of their rights in relation to their personal information.

Across your career, you will encounter new technology designed to support your role, some elements of which you will find more useful than others. Digital literacy skills will enable you to navigate new technology, supporting both colleagues and patients.

Activities: brief outline answers

Activity 5.3

Here are some examples of healthcare data Imani might be collecting from Andrea:

- her nutritional intake through a food and fluid chart;
- her fluid balance;
- her family and next of kin contact information;
- a regular electrocardiogram.

Activity 5.4

Toni's entry is an example of poor record keeping; as a TNA you will know that good-quality records are standards expected from the NMC *Code* (2018a). Poor records could potentially result in deterioration of John's condition and lead to internal investigation, fitness to practise panel and your removal from the NMC register (Brookes, 2021).

An important consideration is the language Toni has used to describe John's personal care. You should avoid using subjective language, that John is 'resistive', which is open to interpretation. In records objectively describe what the behaviour was, and document steps taken to provide care (Brookes, 2021). Poor record keeping is often associated with time, workforce and training barriers. If you feel that record keeping in your organisation does not meet consistent standards, it may be an opportunity to arrange an audit; further information on the audit process in improving care standards will be covered in Chapter 7.

Activity 5.5

Using the EHR to look at an individual health record of someone who is not under your care is against the law and will result in misconduct investigations through the NMC. In 2018 staff members working in a hospital in England were disciplined after accessing singer Ed Sheeran's medical record when he received treatment. The RNA is responsible for ensuring that they 'Respect people's right to privacy and confidentiality' (NMC, 2018a, p. 9). Furthermore, under the Data Protection Act (2018) and GDPR (UK GDPR, 2018) inappropriate use of EHR results is a breach of confidence opening the healthcare organisation and individuals involved to liability. Maintaining the confidentiality of a patient's health information is a fundamental element of professional conduct (Griffith, 2018). You should not be accessing any individual's health record if your use is not justified.

Activity 5.6

Andrea would have had a pressure ulcer risk assessment within the first six hours of her admission to meet Quality Statement 1 of the NICE Quality Standards (2015).

You would use a risk assessment tool, such as a Waterlow scale (2005), to complete the risk assessment within the six-hour time limit.

You would document your assessment, ensuring it's complete, accurate and valid, and sign clearly with your name and role.

Using the data gathered through the Waterlow scale (2005), you would then have a discussion with your team on how to manage Andrea's pressure ulcer risk in accordance with NICE guidelines.

Your timely and accurate assessment and recording of the assessment contributes to retrospective data collected in compliance with the Quality Statement. You might not even know it, but that thorough and timely completed pressure area assessment tool contributes to your unit's recognition as a good service.

Further reading

Health Education England (2019a) *The Topol Review: Preparing the Healthcare Workforce to Deliver the Digital Future*. London: HEE.

The Topol Review is an interesting review into how digital technology can transform healthcare.

Health Education England (2017) *A Health and Care Digital Capabilities Framework*. London: HEE.

A guide to digital skills that will enable healthcare professionals to work within a digital transformation.

Royal College of Nursing (2018) *Every Nurse an E-nurse: Insights from a Consultation on the Digital Future of Nursing*. London: RCN.

This document is a statement from the RCN on digital change in nursing.

Useful websites

Health Education England (n.d.) NHS Digital Academy. Available at: **https://digital-transformation.hee.nhs.uk/digital-academy**

The NHS Digital Academy website has information on projects and learning opportunities for individuals who are interested in the digital transformation of the NHS.

https://digital-transformation.hee.nhs.uk/building-a-digital-workforce/digital-literacy/digital-champions

Provides further information about digital champions.

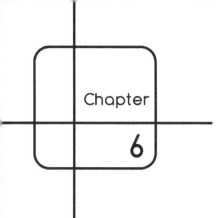

Chapter 6

Understanding prioritisation, workload and delegation

Hazel Cowls

NMC STANDARDS OF PROFICIENCY FOR NURSING ASSOCIATES

This chapter will address the following platforms and proficiencies:

Platform 1: Being an accountable professional

1.1 understand and act in accordance with the Code: Professional standards of practice and behaviour for nurses, midwives and nursing associates, and fulfil all registration requirements.

Platform 3: Provide and monitor care

3.7 demonstrate and apply an understanding of how and when to escalate to the appropriate professional for expert help and advice.

Platform 4: Working in teams

4.1 demonstrate an awareness of the roles, responsibilities and scope of practice of different members of the nursing and interdisciplinary team, and their own role within it.

4.5 demonstrate an ability to prioritise and manage their own workload, and recognise where elements of care can safely be delegated to other colleagues, carers and family members.

Annexe A: Communication and relationship management skills

At the point of registration, the nursing associate will be able to safely demonstrate the following skills:

5. Demonstrate effective supervision skills

Chapter aims

After reading this chapter you will be able to:

- understand the legal, ethical and professional issues that relate to prioritisation and delegation of workload;
- explain how to prioritise work using a matrix or triage system;
- understand the importance of when to delegate workload and how to delegate safely;
- recognise the importance of effective communication to delegate work;
- recognise the barriers to delegation.

Introduction

Trainee and Registered Nursing associates (TNA/RNA) are often in a position where they care for more than one patient, whether this is in a hospital setting, clinic setting or in the community. Being able to effectively prioritise workload and delegate are important leadership skills and, when delegating to others, NAs need to use their critical thinking and decision-making skills to make sure the appropriate course of action is chosen (Standing and Anthony, 2008; Weydt, 2010). The four themes within the Nursing and Midwifery Council (NMC) *Code* (2018a) that underpin your clinical practice are to prioritise people; practice effectively; preserve safety; promote professionalism and trust. When upheld, they ensure good nursing, midwifery and RNA practice that aims to protect the public (NMC, 2018a). The key elements of the Code are to:

- provide compassionate care;
- work collaboratively with the wider team;
- keep accurate records;
- delegate responsibly and to be accountable;
- raise concerns if necessary;
- cooperate with investigations and audit as required (NMC, 2018a).

In this chapter, you will develop your understanding of the legal, ethical and professional issues that relate to prioritisation, workload and delegation (e.g., NMC Standards [2018c] and Royal College of Nursing [RCN]). You will recognise the importance of being able to prioritise work using a matrix or triage system and how this will aid your communication. You will understand the importance of communicating effectively, with sensitivity and compassion, and managing relationships to provide high-quality person-centred care. You will develop your own leadership behaviours and your ability to prioritise and manage your workload as well as recognising where elements of care can be safely delegated to other colleagues, carers and family members.

The legal, ethical and professional issues

Leadership involves managing your workload and that of others, as well as prioritising and delegating work safely. As a leader it is important to understand the legal, ethical and professional principles that underpin our clinical practice. First, we need to understand accountability, responsibility, authority and delegation and you will be familiar with these terms from your own practice and learning. In this section, we will discuss each of these in turn. Accountability is integral to nursing practice and, as an RNA, you are a professional with an assured level of knowledge and skills that enables you to deliver safe effective patient care (NMC, 2018a). We are accountable to ourselves, our patients, our employer and the law. All RNAs must ensure that they work within their level of competence and inform a senior colleague if they are unable to perform competently.

The key functions of accountability in nursing are to prevent negligence and ensure high-quality safe patient care (Griffith and Tengnah, 2017). A brief overview of the four functions of accountability in nursing includes:

1. *protected function*: to protect the public from acts or omissions that may cause harm;
2. *deterrent function*: to always act in a manner worthy of a nurse, in work, public or private. A registrant can be held to account if he/she does not behave appropriately;
3. *regulatory function*: as a registered nurse you are accountable to your patient, your employer and the law. The regulatory framework identifies the standards that you are expected to meet as a registered practitioner;
4. *educational function*: if called to account your behaviour and your practice will be scrutinised, reassuring the public that only the highest standard of practice is accepted. This also allows for others to learn from any mistakes (NMC, 2018c).

All RNAs need to maintain knowledge and skills so that they can confidently explain the rationale for any decisions made. Marquis and Huston (2017) give a broad moralistic view of the term *accountability*, suggesting that any action is deliberate and that the individual is morally responsible for any consequences of actions. As mentioned in Chapter 1, TNAs and RNAs need to be able to demonstrate *contemporary clinical knowledge* – having the knowledge and skills to perform an activity or an intervention. RNAs also need to have the authority to perform an activity in accordance with local policies and procedures, as well as be responsible for completing the activity. This is important and relevant to nursing practice as it ensures that RNAs are working in accordance with the NMC *Code* and the law.

Responsibility is allocated and, once accepted, implies ownership; in nursing it is about being able to perform specific skills and duties or make decisions. For example, if a TNA or RNA is allocated a task to complete a urinalysis test, they are responsible for ensuring the results are documented clearly, and that they report any abnormality as per local policy and procedures. As a trainee or RNA, you are also responsible for continuous self-reflection, seeking and gaining feedback from others so that you may develop your professional knowledge and skills (NMC, 2018b).

Authority refers to the right to act in areas of given and accepted responsibility. There are various levels of authority ranging from gathering information to making decisions, recommendations, initiating actions and delegating. *Delegation* is defined as the action or process of delegating or being delegated. It is about entrusting or committing others to complete a task: for example, a TNA may delegate completing a set of clinical observations on an individual to a healthcare assistant. The TNA is delegating responsibility and authority to a specified person to complete the assigned task, but is accountable for that decision to delegate.

When *prioritising* workload and delegating we need to be mindful of the ethical principles described by Beauchamp and Childress (2013) as follows:

- *respect for autonomy*: to value the individual right to make a choice;
- *non-maleficence*: to do no harm and prevent harm;
- *justice*: to act fairly and with justice to patients/service users;
- *beneficence*: to act with goodness for the well-being of patients/service users.

Marquis and Huston (2017) expanded on these principles by adding *paternalism*, the right to decide for another; *utility*, that the good of many outweighs the rights of one individual; *veracity*, to be honest; and, finally, the *need to keep promises*. Examples of each of these principles are shown in Table 6.1.

Table 6.1 Examples illustrating ethical principles

Paternalism	A doctor may decide that a decision is not in the best interest for a 20-year-old woman to have a sterilisation.
Utility	Clinical commissioning group deciding upon a treatment that can be offered to 50 patients in comparison to treating one person.
Veracity	The TNA informs a patient that a repeat blood sample is required as the first sample haemolysed.
Fidelity	The TNA informs a young patient that she will return in 30 minutes, and she does return within the time stated.

How to prioritise work?

Prioritisation of work is about managing your workload effectively and ensuring tasks are completed. The workload may differ from person to person depending upon your role – for example, you may be a manager who needs to coordinate the work of a team or an RNA or a TNA delivering a clinic or managing a caseload of patients in the community. When prioritising workload, there are various things that you may need to consider, such as:

- how many tasks you need to complete;
- what is urgent and what is important (see Table 6.2);
- the level of urgency to complete the task(s), such as patient need or whether there is a deadline to submit a report;

- what resources are available to you to help you complete the task(s);
- whether you can delegate any work safely to another person (we will look at delegation in more detail later in the chapter).

Table 6.2   Time management matrix

	URGENT	**NOT URGENT**
IMPORTANT	Prioritise	Add to the 'to do list'
NOT IMPORTANT	Delegate	Remove from the 'to do list'

Source: Adapted from the 'time management matrix' (Covey, 1989), also known as Eisenhower matrix.

The time management or Eisenhower matrix is a task management tool to aid prioritisation of work. It is called the 'Eisenhower' matrix after President Eisenhower (34th President of the United States), who developed this principle as he needed to make important decisions daily. The matrix is split into four quadrants with each quadrant being classified as urgent/not urgent and important/not important. In the first quadrant, a task that is both urgent and important, such as a patient in cardiac arrest, needs to be prioritised. In the second quadrant, a task such as completing a routine medicine (drug) round is important but may not be urgent. Transferring a patient to another ward is a good example of a task in the third quadrant as it is urgent but may not be important so this task could be delegated. Finally, in the fourth quadrant, making a stationery order could be classed as neither urgent nor important and could be removed from the list.

Activity 6.1   Reflection

We can apply the principles of the time management matrix to all aspects of our life whether personal or professional.

You may have a list of things that you need to complete. Can you apply the time management matrix to your own life? Draw up your own time management matrix.

As this activity is based on your own observation, there is no outline answer at the end of the chapter.

Prioritising workload involves decision-making, so what is decision-making? We begin the process of decision-making during childhood and this continues throughout our personal and professional life. Each day we analyse situations, create solutions to problems, make choices, act upon decisions. Banning (2008) suggested that clinical decision-making is about choosing one course of action over all other options, and it is a skill that improves through experience. However, deciding upon one course of action means rejecting other options and may be associated with consequences or feelings of regret. Remember, the more choices that you must consider, the more skilful you need to become to make the choice.

So, what helps us to make decisions? Factors that aid clinical decision-making include learning from experience, reflective practice, developing knowledge and skills, logical thinking and an awareness of any bias such as unconscious bias. *Unconscious bias* is defined as: 'an unfair belief about a group of people that you are not aware of and that affects your behaviour and decisions' (*Oxford Learner's Dictionary*, n.d.).

Decision-making requires critical thinking; this is defined as the practice of analysing and considering all aspects of a situation and the evidence about what works best when making decisions (NMC, 2018c; Peate, 2019). The following resources may influence our decision-making:

- *facts*: taken from patient notes such as a clinical history or test results;
- *knowledge*: theoretical knowledge, professional regulations, clinical guidelines, policies and procedures, ethical and legal considerations, knowledge of people and their circumstances;
- *experience*: professional regulations, experiential knowledge, discipline, multidisciplinary team;
- *analysis*: undertaken before a judgement is made and can be objective or subjective;
- *judgement*: a combination of the above but also includes clinical risk (Mok and Stevens, 2005).

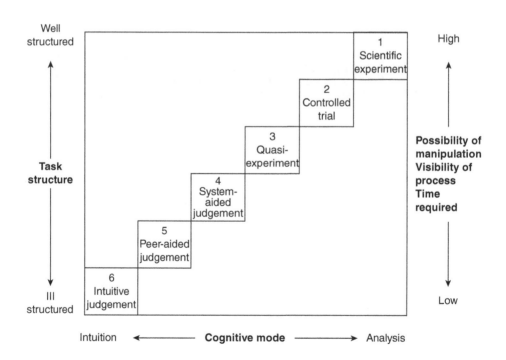

Figure 6.1   Cognitive Continuum Theory

Source: Hamm (1988), reproduced with kind permission of Cambridge University Press.

In practice, a healthcare professional may be required to make rapid clinical decisions under uncertain conditions such as in an emergency setting. Any decision-making may be influenced by both objective and subjective data available at the time, as well as the RNA's understanding of the data, their knowledge base and perception of the problem presented. Cognitive Continuum Theory (CCT) illustrates how specific judgements or tasks relate to cognition (Hammond, 1981). Hammond (1981) identified six *modes of enquiry* ranging from unrestricted judgement to analytical judgement. These were replaced with six *modes of practice* (Hamm, 1988) – see Figure 6.1. These have been shown to aid clinical decision-making in medicine and in nursing (Thompson, 1999) by helping nurses explain their rationale for decisions made.

CCT is useful as it helps all nurses to develop their analytical skills in order to make clinical decisions. Decisions 1–4 above are based on empirical evidence – that is, systematic reviews, research and audit (analytical judgement), whereas decisions 5–6 are based on experience and intuition (intuitive judgement) (Gopee and Galloway, 2017). Hamm (1988) suggests that the intuitive judgement is often made when the task is complex, unfamiliar and time is limited, whereas tasks that are well structured such as analysing test results require analysis and can be broken down into smaller components.

Case study: Judgements

1. *An analytical judgement*

   Georgina is a TNA looking after a sixteen-week-old baby who has been admitted with projectile vomiting. Georgina records a high temperature of 37.8°C; mum reports her baby has been breathless when feeding and does not appear to be gaining any weight. As a TNA Georgina recognises the importance of this new information and reports to the nurse in charge and the paediatrician. Georgina is aware that further tests may be required for this baby but is not sure what tests the paediatrician will request. However, the tests will build a clinical picture to aid decision-making. This is an example of analytical judgement seen in clinical practice.

2. *Intuitive judgement*

   Simon is a TNA. He sees an elderly patient in a GP waiting room who is looking pale and holding his chest. Simon's intuitive thought is that the patient may be experiencing a heart attack and he needs to act quickly. Given Simon's experience and knowledge this task is complex, unfamiliar and timely. As a TNA he will need to assess the patient, reassure the patient, call for help and act quickly. This is an example of intuitive judgement seen in clinical practice.

The more experienced professional may be inclined to use intuition and peer-aided judgement (Benner, 2001[1984]; Pretz and Folse, 2010) to make informed decisions. However, using intuition and peer-aided judgement in nursing could be seen as controversial and be viewed as less scientific and not valid. Have you ever heard a colleague say 'I have a gut feeling' about a patient's condition? The experiences that lead to intuition, or a 'gut feeling' are often more than intuition – based on pattern recognition, prior experience and knowledge and critical thinking, as well as evidence (Melin-Johannson et al., 2017).

We know that prioritising care leads to safe, effective patient care but at times can challenge nurses' moral and professional values. Suhonen et al. (2018) stated that prioritising for nurses is difficult, with nurses reporting moral distress and missed care that affected patient outcomes, as well as nursing professional practice and quality of care compromise. Gopee and Galloway (2017) suggest the following good practice guidelines for effective decision-making and problem-solving:

- accept decision-making and see it as a learning opportunity for positive learning outcomes;
- do not delay any decision-making as this may lead to complications;
- use a systematic approach to decision-making whenever possible;
- set clear goals when making decisions;
- allow individuals and teams time and space to develop creativity when facing any challenges.

Applying decision-making to clinical practice

In general practice and in a hospital environment, prioritising patients is known as *triage*. The word comes from the French verb *trier*, meaning to sort or select. Although triage is commonly used in emergency healthcare, it can be broken down into three phases: pre-hospital, at the scene of the event and emergency department triage. There are numerous tools used in clinical practice to aid triage, but the universal goal is to standardise the assessment of a person's needs, prioritise their care and identify who is best placed to offer evidence-based care (Royal College of Physicians [RCP], 2017). EConsult® is an example of an online triage and consultation system where patients can access self-help resources as well as access medical advice. The system was first introduced in primary care in the UK in the early 2000s and then rolled out as part of the *NHS Long Term Plan* to improve patient access to services by offering e-consultations in the UK (NHS England, 2019). This plan was accelerated in 2020 to reduce the contagion of Covid-19. This shift to remote consultation has been successful, with telephone consulting being sufficient for most patients, and SMS-messaging increasing more than three-fold (Murphy et al., 2021).

In the emergency care setting triage is a brief intervention that usually occurs within fifteen minutes of presentation to the department (Royal College of Emergency Medicine, 2017). Triage staff are registered practitioners that are appropriately trained and experienced in emergency care. Following a clinical assessment (to include a patient history and obtaining vital signs) the patient will be allocated to a group or an area in the department where they will be seen by the right practitioner. The clinician or nurse will often use an early warning system such as National Early Warning System (NEWS) to assess a patient's clinical condition and ascertain how quickly a person's care may need escalating. You may already be familiar with NEWS scoring, which is based on a simple aggregate scoring system; a score is allocated to six physiological measurements (respiration rate, oxygen saturation, systolic blood pressure, pulse rate, level of consciousness or new confusion, temperature) (RCP, 2017).

In 2017, the Royal College of Paediatrics and Child Health, NHS England and the RCN collaborated to develop a Paediatric Early Warning System (PEWS) in England; following the roll-out of a PEWS in Scotland, Northern Ireland and Ireland there have been calls to make this nationwide. The PEWS is a 'track and trigger' tool used to identify a deteriorating child or young person in primary, secondary and tertiary care. A review of a sample of PEWS charts used across the UK highlighted great variation in practice, such as: a variation in which parameters contribute to the score; whether blood pressure is included in the score; how to record behavioural change and parental concern; different charts used to account for the change in child's physiology between birth and adulthood (Roland et al., 2021).

In the emergency department people are triaged on arrival at the hospital. Figure 6.2 gives an example of triage, where patients are identified as a specific priority group depending upon their presentation (description). For instance, a patient who presents with a life-threatening injury in the pre-hospital or emergency department phase needs emergency/immediate care.

Priority Group			
Number	Name	Color	Description
P1	Emergency/Immediate	Red	Patients who have life-threatening injuries that are treatable with a minimum amount of time, personnel, and supplies. These patients also have a good chance of recovery.
P2	Urgent	Yellow	Indicates that treatment may be delayed for a limited period of time without significant mortality or in the ICU setting patients for whom life support may or may not change their outcome given the severity of their illness.
P3	Delayed	Green	Patients with minor injuries whose treatment may be delayed until the patients in the other categories have been dealt with or patients who do not require ICU admission for the provision of life support.
P4	Expectant	Blue	Patients who have injuries requiring extensive treatment that exceeds the medical resources available in the situation or for whom life support is considered futile.
–	Dead	Black	Patients who are in cardiac arrest and for which resuscitation efforts are not going to be provided.

Figure 6.2   Priority groups commonly used in triage for health care

Source: Christian (2019), reproduced by kind permission of Elsevier.

The following case study will illustrate clinical decision-making and how to prioritise care.

Case study: Prioritising caseload

Michael is a second-year TNA working with a community nursing team. Today, Michael is working with a third-year nursing student, Jay, and they are planning their workload for the day. They have received two telephone referrals requesting their input.

(Continued)

(Continued)

Referral 1: Yuri is an elderly gentleman who lives alone in a ground-floor flat. He has reported low abdominal pain overnight and poor sleep. He is known to have an indwelling catheter in situ. Yuri sounded muddled on the telephone. Yuri lives six miles away from the community nurse office.

Referral 2: Elizabeth is 60 years old and lives with her husband. She has recently been in hospital for a primary elective knee replacement. Elizabeth was seen by a physiotherapist pre-discharge for rehabilitation and has been shown relevant strengthening exercises. Upon discharge from hospital, Elizabeth was informed that she would be seen by the community nurse two days post discharge to check her wound and that she may need a dressing change. Elizabeth lives a mile away from the community nurse office.

Activity 6.2   In practice

Michael and Jay need to decide which patient to see first but they have received limited information. It is important to gather as much information as possible before making any clinical decisions. Decision-making is a complex, cognitive process that involves gathering information, analysing and evaluating information before making a clinical judgement and deciding a course of action (Marquis and Huston, 2017).

Which patient do they see first and why?

An outline answer is given at the end of this chapter.

Why and how do we delegate?

Let us look at a typical clinical environment where the team have arrived for a day shift and have allocated their workload. The team are responsible for a group of patients and need to ensure that patients have appropriate care such as administering their medication on time, arranging referrals to other healthcare professionals (HCPs) and arranging a patient transfer to another hospital, as well as ensuring a member of the nursing team attends the ward round and helps arrange discharges. An HCP calls a TNA over to see a person urgently, but the TNA needs to make referrals to other HCPs; how do they ensure that all the patients' needs are addressed? It is likely that some of the workload will need to be delegated to another colleague. The NMC (2018c) suggests that there are three reasons why we delegate:

1. to ensure that the people we are looking after getting the care that they need;
2. to ensure students have opportunities to develop their clinical skills;
3. to ensure patients and families are involved in care.

Registered nurses, midwives and NAs are accountable for any decisions made around delegation. As a registered nurse, midwife, or NA, you must only delegate work that is within another person's scope of competence, including having an understanding of the activity; that the person to who you have delegated work is well supported and supervised if necessary; and that you confirm the outcome of any activity delegated (NMC, 2018a).

Delegating work poorly can result in poor patient outcomes, so nurses need to ensure that they are knowledgeable, competent and confident in their decisions (Standing and Anthony, 2008). The RCN suggests that the underlying principles of delegation are:

1. to ensure that delegating activities is always in the best interest of the patient;
2. to ensure the support worker has been suitably trained to perform the activities or intervention;
3. to ensure the support worker has access to ongoing development to ensure competency is maintained;
4. to ensure that all records of staff competence are recorded and dates of training given are documented;
5. all staff have access to clear guidelines and protocols are in place;
6. all delegated activities are within the support worker's job description;
7. the person who delegates any activity must ensure that an appropriate level of supervision is available to the support worker. The level of supervision will depend upon the knowledge and competence of the support worker as well as the needs of the patient/client, the activities or care assigned and the clinical setting;
8. any risks are identified.

As mentioned above, delegating work can help others to develop their skills and it can promote team-working. As a team leader or manager, you will want to ensure that the work is completed to an acceptable standard but at times it can be difficult to relinquish a task. The *five rights* of delegation can assist nurses in making safe decisions around delegation; these are:

- right task;
- right circumstance;
- right person;
- right supervision;
- right direction and communication (Neumann, 2010).

Case study: Johanna, part 1

Five rights of delegation

Johanna is a second-year TNA and is working a night shift on a twenty-bedded elder care rehabilitation ward. During a busy shift Johanna has several tasks to complete, including: changing bed linen, as a patient has been incontinent; seeing a

(Continued)

(Continued)

patient who has just reported pain; and completing a care round. Johanna needs to delegate some work to colleagues and will use the five rights of delegation to help with decision-making.

Right task

Johanna needs to determine which tasks are right to delegate and will need to consider local policies and procedures before making any decisions. For example, it would not be appropriate to delegate care of a person in pain to an unregistered colleague as the patient may require analgesia.

Right circumstance

Next Johanna may need to consider whether there are appropriate resources available to delegate a task: does the delegatee have the right skills and is supervision required? For example, if a person is at risk of seizures, then it would not be appropriate to delegate care to an unregistered colleague.

Right person

Next Johanna needs to consider whether the delegatee has prior knowledge, experience and skills to complete the task. Johanna may need to ask whether the delegatee has completed any specific training and whether this task is within their scope of practice and job description.

Right supervision

After establishing the right task, right circumstance and right person, Johanna needs to check whether supervision is required? This ensures the task is completed safely. Johanna must ensure that the delegatee provides feedback once the task is completed. Providing constructive feedback on a person's skills, knowledge and behaviour, including what they think went well and where improvements could be made, is important (NMC, 2018a).

Right direction and communication

Johanna must give clear instructions to the delegatee, so that the delegatee understands the task and reports back once the task is completed.

By applying the five rights of delegation, you are demonstrating an understanding of the legal, ethical and professional issues that relate to prioritisation and delegation of workload. Each of these 'rights' are equally important but giving the right direction and communication can minimise any misunderstandings within the team and reduce any conflict. We will discuss communication in more detail later in the chapter. Remember that as TNA you need to recognise where elements of care can be safely delegated to other health and social care professionals, carers and their families (NMC, 2018b).

Activity 6.3   Reflection

You have read about why we delegate; please list the types of duties or activities that you delegate to others or could delegate to others.

Identify to whom you do, or could, delegate activities ?

What factors do you need to consider when delegating an activity?

An outline answer is given at the end of this chapter.

RNAs play an active role within the interdisciplinary team and work collaboratively to ensure that care is delivered safely (NMC, 2018b). Interdisciplinary team-working is discussed in more detail in Chapter 3. RNAs need to be able to manage their own workload, prioritise cases and delegate care if indicated (NMC, 2018b, 4.5). In a recent qualitative study based at a large healthcare organisation, NAs discussed how the acquisition of knowledge and critical thinking would enable them to work more independently and with increased responsibility (Lucas et al., 2021). The following case illustrates the prioritisation of workload, leadership and team-working.

Case study: Johanna, part 2

Johanna has returned to the community hospital placement. The ward is a twenty-bedded elder care rehabilitation ward accepting both male and female patients. Unfortunately, half the ward is closed as there has been an increase in cases of Covid affecting both patients and staff. The ward manager has contacted a nursing agency to arrange cover and ensure there are enough registered and unregistered staff on duty. The day staff arrive on duty and, apart from Johanna, only one newly registered nurse (NRN) is a permanent member of staff – with all other staff being agency workers and not familiar with the ward. Other staff working on the ward include a Foundation Year 1 doctor (F1), ancillary staff such as the ward domestic, ward clerk and kitchen assistant. Johanna is allocated a bay of patients to look after, and notices that one patient is showing signs of Covid (new continuous cough, short of breath and reports a headache) (NHS, 2022b). Johanna arranges for the patient to complete a lateral flow test and this confirms that the patient is Covid-positive. Johanna informs the NRN, the nurse in charge of the patient lateral flow results, and waits for instructions. The NRN is also new to the ward and looked to the team for advice on how to manage the possible outbreak of Covid. Johanna is familiar with the hospital's local policy and procedures and, specifically, the hospital policy for the management of a suspected or confirmed outbreak of Covid.

Activity 6.4   Critical thinking

Thinking about this case, how can Johanna manage this scenario? What skills does Johanna need to employ to ensure that the situation is managed well?

If you have been involved in a similar situation, take some time to reflect on that situation. What happened, what did you do, what went well and what could be improved?

An outline answer is given at the end of this chapter.

In Part 2 of the case study, Johanna (TNA) knew the team and knew who she could draw on to help manage the situation; therefore, she was able to delegate work to different people.

Due to the global pandemic, we have seen changes in how health and social care services are delivered that have included people working differently, such as online consultations, telephone assessments and people diversifying within their role. A recent study looking at the impact of Covid-19 on work and well-being concluded that there was a noticeable change in working practices for TNAs, such as substituting for staff shortages, taking on cleaning duties to support infection, prevention and control and broadening their scope of practice (King et al., 2021). Prior to Covid-19 TNAs and RNAs reported a lack of clarity about their role (Davey, 2019; King et al., 2021) and this was exacerbated by Covid-19 due to the change in practices, although some TNAs enjoyed the challenge of extending their scope of practice (King et al., 2021). Despite the stressors reported in clinical practice brought about due to Covid-19, TNAs did report improved team-working and a sense of connection with colleagues, as well as patients and their relatives (King et al., 2021). Health and social care provision is an area that is constantly changing according to the needs of our communities and funding and, as healthcare professionals, we need to be able to move with the changing environment.

Activity 6.5   Critical thinking

Thinking about delegation in action, make a list of what you think the positives and negatives might be.

An outline answer is given at the end of this chapter.

In summary, delegating workload can have a positive impact on individuals, patients and their families, as well as the organisation. Delegating work can create opportunities for people to develop, lead to increased job satisfaction and may lead to retention of staff. However, delegation can also lead to conflict within teams and avoidance of work which will have a negative impact on the organisational environment.

The importance of communication

Earlier in the chapter you were introduced to the five rights of delegation; the fifth right is direction and communication. You will have previously studied communication and be aware that there are several models and definitions of communication, but, in its simplest form, communication is when one person transmits a message in some form to another person (Webb, 2020). You will understand that communicating effectively with sensitivity and compassion is essential to providing high-quality safe patient care (NMC, 2018b). At times this can be challenging; as health and social care providers, we work in a high-pressure profession and there are many factors that can contribute to this pressure. In recent years we have seen increasing demands being placed on health and social care professionals which can only increase the level of distress people may be experiencing. Pierre et al. (2007) identified the following reasons why communication is complex in acute care, although these reasons could be applied to any clinical setting:

- uncertainty;
- information overload;
- time pressures;
- multiple goals and priorities;
- multiple people involved.

Other factors that may inhibit effective communication are working alongside people that you do not necessarily like, misunderstanding what you have been asked to do, not appreciating each other's workload, not recognising the skills required to complete tasks, not recognising whether a colleague requires supervision. All these factors can contribute to conflict in teams and may inhibit patient care.

In Chapter 3 you were introduced to the concept of communicating with compassion. If you are to apply the four elements of compassionate communication as described by West (2021), such as paying attention to other people, demonstrating understanding and empathy when a person may be feeling overworked or stressed and offering to help where possible, then this may help mitigate any negative feelings between teams.

Understanding the theory: compassionate communication

1. Paying attention to the other person – *attending*.
2. Understanding what is causing the other person distress – *understanding*.
3. Being empathetic by mirroring the other person's feelings – *empathising*.
4. Taking intelligent action to help relieve any suffering – *helping*.

As a TNA you will need to demonstrate effective communication skills when working in teams, including giving clear instructions and checking understanding when delegating care responsibilities to others, as well as providing constructive feedback (NMC, 2018b).

The way a team member is asked to perform an activity by the delegating TNA is likely to influence the team-worker's response. For example, compare the two examples below as Ramil (TNA) requests that a colleague (Alicia) completes a task.

Option 1. Ramil telephones Alicia with a request to complete task A within one hour and then Ramil ends the telephone call.

Option 2. Ramil telephones Alicia with a request to complete task A. Ramil gives clear instructions on what needs to be done and checks that Alicia understands her role and the task; she checks that Alicia has the necessary skills and time to complete the task. Ramil and Alicia agree a timeframe for the task to be completed. Ramil requests that Alicia informs him when she has completed the task.

Option 1 is an autocratic approach and there appears to be no consideration for Alicia's time or knowledge and skills to complete the task. Ramil is not communicating with compassion. In option 2, however, Ramil is being democratic as he is negotiating with Alicia and involving her in the decision-making. It is highly likely that Alicia is going to be more responsive to option 2 as this option is polite, respectful and ensures safe practice.

Understanding the theory: competence and motivation

In Chapter 2 you explored leadership theories and styles, and you will recognise that different approaches in leadership are necessary, depending upon the circumstances. For example, in a clinical emergency an appropriate approach may be directing or coaching as the leader is concerned with specific task accomplishment or policies and procedures rather than developing relations with the team. Contingency theorists such as Fieldler (in the late 1960s) and Hersey et al. (2001) suggest that the most effective leadership style is one that complements the person, the task and the organisation, so different situations require different approaches.

Table 6.3 illustrates difference leadership approaches used depending on the individual's level of competence and motivation. For example, a first-year TNA who has completed some initial training on wound care and therefore possesses some competence may require *coaching* to complete the patient care. In contrast, a second-year TNA who is managing a ward may *delegate* workload to colleagues.

Table 6.3 Individual level of competence and motivation for tasks

Individual level of competence/motivation	Appropriate leadership style
1. Low competence/high commitment	Directing
2. Some competence/low commitment	Coaching
3. High competence/variable commitment	Supporting
4. High competence/high commitment	Delegating

Source: Adapted from Hersey et al., 2001.

Activity 6.6 Communication

You have explored individuals' levels of competence and motivation. Using Hersey et al.'s (2001) situational leadership model please match the following person and scenario with the appropriate leadership style:

Person/activity

First-year NA – changing a wound dressing

Healthcare assistant – just completed the observation course

Family member – wishing to learn how to change a dressing for a family member

First-year NA – day one on a ward

House-keeping staff – not completing fluid and food charts properly

Leadership style

Directing

Coaching

Supporting

Delegating

An outline answer is given at the end of this chapter.

Good communication skills that include listening and understanding will lead to good team-working, effective delegation and safe patient care. Throughout your clinical practice you will be directing, coaching, supporting and delegating work to others within your team. The final case study and activity below illustrates delegation in clinical practice.

Case study: Delegation

Paul is a second-year TNA and is working with Anya, who is a first-year TNA and has just started a placement in your practice area, which is an acute medical ward. Anya informs Paul that she has attended clinical skills at university, has practised taking clinical observations and feels confident to take patient clinical observations. Mr Jansons has been admitted to your ward and is known to have a condition called atrial fibrillation (an irregular heartbeat); because of this irregular heartbeat manual observations need to be carried out as the electronic equipment may not record an accurate pulse or blood pressure. Paul asks Anya to make sure all the observations are taken manually. Paul shows Anya where the equipment is located. However, ten minutes later Paul notices that Anya is placing the electronic monitoring on the patient and seems flustered.

Reviewing the case study above, please answer the following questions:

1.   What should Paul do and why?
2.   Which leadership style would be appropriate for Paul to use?
3.   How would Paul manage the situation for the patient and Anya?

An outline answer is given at the end of this chapter.

Understanding the barriers to good delegation

Throughout this chapter we have looked at how to and why we delegate, but it is also important to understand the barriers to delegation. Although nurses recognise that delegation is an important part of leadership, some nurses do not feel confident to delegate work and end up completing the work themselves rather than asking for help (Trueland, 2021). Some nurse leaders or managers may be reluctant to delegate work because they are not confident that anyone can complete the task to their standard, but this may just be their own perception. If the leader has not asked anyone, how do they know that the task cannot be completed to their standard? There may not be anyone in the team with the right knowledge and skills to complete a task, but through the appraisal process a leader could identify people to develop their knowledge and skills. Some leaders may not delegate work because they are worried that someone within the team may complete a task better than them and this may be about their own feeling of worth in the team. Some leaders report that it would be quicker for them to complete the task themselves rather than delegating to another and having to explain or teach the task.

Delegation can also be done poorly – for example, not being clear about what needs to be done or why, may lead to a *no-win situation* where it is unlikely the delegatee would complete the task; or delegating a task that you do not like doing yourself (Trueland, 2021). Either way there is a risk that poor delegation could be used maliciously – for example, delegating a task to someone you may not like, leading to accusations around bullying or harassment. The consequences of not delegating well or just not delegating are as follows:

1.   the leader or manager may experience *burn out* (chronic workplace stress) due to feeling overworked and work-related stress;
2.   staff may not feel valued in the workplace and this may lead to conflict in the team or staff leaving the workplace;
3.   staff are not able to develop their knowledge and skills and, as registered nurses, midwives and NAs, it is important that staff have opportunities to develop professionally;
4.   possible conflict in the team;
5.   poor retention and recruitment of staff.

The first step to breaking down these barriers to delegation is recognising that there is an issue and then working with team members and leaders to explore each barrier.

Chapter summary

This chapter has explored the legal, ethical and professional issues that relate to prioritisation and delegation of workload and how this will support your practice. According to the NMC, there are three core reasons why we delegate: to ensure people are receiving the care that they need; to ensure that students have opportunities to develop their skills; and to ensure that patients and families are involved in their care. You will need to consider these in your own clinical practice. Prioritising and delegating work can be challenging at times and may lead to misunderstandings or conflict within teams. However, we have discussed the importance of communicating with compassion through effective listening, understanding, empathising and helping others. This chapter helps you to understand that by applying the nine principles of delegation you and your colleagues are working within your scope of practice. This chapter has also presented various clinical tools that will help you to make the right clinical decisions such as the time management matrix, five rights of delegation and track and trigger tools (NEWS or PEWS).

Activities: brief outline answers

Activity 6.2

In this case study it would be appropriate to telephone each patient to gather more information so that you can assess the level of urgency and importance of each visit. Yuri reported significant pain and is known to have previously experienced problems with the indwelling urinary catheter blocking. Elizabeth stated that she was just chasing up her appointment as suggested by the hospital discharge team, she reports a low level of pain and is not unduly worried about her wound dressing. Therefore, by applying the time management matrix, Yuri needs to be seen first as his case is both urgent and important compared to Elizabeth's case which is important but not urgent.

Activity 6.3

The list of duties or activities that you delegate to others will be personal to your clinical practice. Examples include:

- taking a blood pressure recording;
- taking a blood sample;
- transferring a patient to another ward or department;

- gathering documentation;
- referring to another agency or professional.

Depending upon the task you could delegate up or down (to a registered nurse, doctor, healthcare assistant, allied healthcare professional). The factors that you need to consider when delegating a task are as follows:

- the reasons for the delegation are understood;
- the expected timeframe and outcome are understood;
- the authority and resources to see the task through are in place;
- the recipient of the delegated task has the necessary support;
- feedback is provided on the results of the delegation.

Activity 6.4

This scenario relates to NMC (2018b), Platforms 1 and 4. As Johanna is familiar with the local trust policies it would be appropriate for her to take the lead on this scenario. As there is a mixed team of people caring for the adult patients, Johanna will need to delegate workload to registered practitioners as well as unqualified staff such as HCPs and ancillary workers. The infection, prevention and control team (IPAC) will need to be informed as they are monitoring all outbreaks of Covid. Patients will need to be isolated, so it is likely that the cleaning staff may need to be involved and patients' families will also need to be informed. It is possible that there will be a change in the visiting policy so relevant people such as the hospital switchboard will also need to be informed. Johanna is acting as the leader and delegating work so she will need to have an awareness of who is completing each task as well as the skill set of each person. For example, a registered nurse or Johanna could speak with the IPAC team and the ward clerk could start telephoning patient families. The skills required to manage this situation include:

- sound knowledge of the policy and procedures;
- good communication with the multidisciplinary team;
- good listening skills as staff or patients may express concerns;
- confidence to lead others;
- ability to delegate work safely.

Activity 6.5

The positives to delegation include:

- opportunities for staff development;
- increased job satisfaction;
- increased motivation and self-esteem;
- positive organisational culture;
- develops leadership qualities;
- enables team leaders to develop staff.

The negatives to delegation include:

- if the person that the task is delegated to is not competent at the task;
- conflict between team members;
- avoidance of work or tasks;
- miscommunication between team members.

Activity 6.6

First-year NA: changing a wound dressing	*Supporting or delegating*
Healthcare assistant: just completed the observation course	*Directing or coaching*
Family member: wishing to learn how to change a dressing for a family member	*Directing*
First-year NA: day one on a ward	*Directing or coaching*
House-keeping staff: not completing fluid and food charts properly	*Directing*

Activity 6.7

This scenario relates to NMC (2018b) Platform 4 and Appendix A, demonstrating effective supervision skills. Recording and documenting an accurate blood pressure and pulse is essential for safe patient care. It would be advisable for Paul to speak to Anya quietly to ascertain their competence and confidence in undertaking these skills. If Anya does not feel competent then Paul may need to complete the task or delegate to someone else who is competent. A transactional or autocratic style would be appropriate as this is about patient safety. However, a transformational leadership style would also work as this would be viewed as supportive. The skills that Paul could apply are directing or coaching skills. It would be beneficial for Paul to arrange a practice session in obtaining manual observations; this could include other members of the team.

Further reading

NHS Leadership Academy learning hub. Available at: **learninghub.leadership academy.nhs.uk /all-bitesize/**

This is a series of short courses to help you to build your knowledge and skills. The bitesize learning will cover topics such as courageous conversations, making decisions under pressure and resilience. You will need to register and log in to access the free resources.

Useful websites

https://econsult.net

eConsult is an online consultation platform that asks specific questions to enable healthcare professionals to triage and prioritise care, ensuring people have access to appropriate self-care resources or an appointment is scheduled.

The NMC has provided two short videos on accountability and delegation:

www.nmc.org.uk/standards/code/code-in-action/accountability/

Accountability: A short video that illustrates being accountable, held to account for your actions and able to confidently explain how you used your professional judgement to make decisions.

www.nmc.org.uk/standards/code/code-in-action/delegation/

Delegation: A short video that illustrates how to delegate.

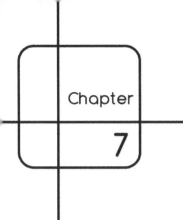

Chapter

7

Understanding how to monitor and review quality of care

Natalie Cusack

NMC STANDARDS OF PROFICIENCY FOR NURSING ASSOCIATES

This chapter will address the following platforms and proficiencies:

Platform 1: Being an accountable professional

1.2 understand and apply relevant legal, regulatory and governance requirements, policies, and ethical frameworks, including any mandatory reporting duties, to all areas of practice.

1.4 demonstrate an understanding of, and the ability to, challenge or report discriminatory behaviour.

1.12 recognise and report any factors that may adversely impact safe and effective care provision.

Platform 5: Improving safety and quality of care

5.2 participate in data collection to support audit activity, and contribute to the implementation of quality improvement strategies.

5.5 recognise when inadequate staffing levels impact on the ability to provide safe care and escalate concerns appropriately.

5.6 understand and act in line with local and national organisational frameworks, legislation and regulations to report risks, and implement actions as instructed, following up and escalating as required.

Chapter aims

After reading this chapter you will be able to:

* define what 'quality' of care means in health and identify guidelines, frameworks and regulatory bodies that guide us to deliver quality care;

(Continued)

(Continued)

- understand the process of audit, patient feedback and peer feedback for monitoring good practice;
- be confident in challenging poor care within your team, advocating for patients and their families;
- be confident in raising risk incidents, safeguarding and whistle-blowing when care falls below standard.

Introduction

Over the previous chapters you have been introduced to the concept of leadership and your responsibilities as a leader in health. In this chapter we will explore the role of a nursing associate in monitoring the quality of services to deliver safe and effective care, aiming for excellent patient experience and satisfaction. This topic is essential in contemporary healthcare; good leadership, with the ability to challenge poor care and advocate for patients, prevents unacceptable events such as Mid-Staffordshire, Winterbourne View and the recent Edenfield Centre investigation prompted by a report from BBC's *Panorama* in 2022.

The common themes within these shocking examples are leadership and management failure to address negative culture (DoH, 2012; Francis, 2013), poor quality of care, such as basic physical needs not being addressed (DoH, 2012), and, in the case of Mid-Staffordshire, noticeable staff shortages and 'assumptions that monitoring, performance management or interventions was the responsibility of someone else' (Francis, 2013, p. 4).

As is made clear in the NMC *Code* (2018a), it is everyone's responsibility to monitor care quality and escalate concerns when appropriate. As you finish your training and work in practice, you may be faced with difficult situations, understaffing, limited resources and negative media coverage of your profession. No one enters the nursing profession with the intention of giving poor care to patients and their families or carers, but we know poor care does happen across the UK. This chapter aims to equip you with an understanding of what good-quality care looks like, regulatory bodies that set standards and, finally, how to monitor and challenge poor care within your workplace, taking necessary steps to document and raise issues to be addressed.

Activity 7.1   Reflection

Reflecting on the time you have spent as a TNA, patient or if a loved one has received care, create a list of what you would expect from the best-quality healthcare service.

You may want to revisit this list over the chapter. Are your wants and needs reflected in standards that we follow?

As your list will be personal to you and your experiences, there are no answers provided.

What is quality? Standards and regulatory bodies

To deliver excellent care, we first need to explore what defines 'quality' in healthcare, the standards we adhere to and who holds responsibility for monitoring health service providers and the people who work there. *Quality* is when goods or a service meets an expectation of standards, across the UK; health services should meet a standard of care that is safe, clinically effective and maximises the patient experience (National Quality Board, 2013).

Case study: James

To visualise quality in action, let's imagine the patient journey for James, a 50-year-old man who attends accident and emergency experiencing chest pain and breathlessness.

Safe: James is seen by a triage nurse who completes an assessment and refers him to the correct hospital department; he is risk assessed and monitored for deterioration. All staff who meet James follow infection control procedures to avoid passing on hospital-acquired infection and the equipment used to monitor James' condition is clean and maintained regularly with in-date safety certificates.

Clinically effective: James is monitored according to national clinical guidelines for adults presenting with acute chest pain (NICE, 2016). He receives diagnostic tests, such as an electrocardiogram, by staff who are appropriately trained. James is prescribed oxygen and medication to relieve his symptoms. His nursing team monitor his physical observation at regular intervals using evidence-based early warning systems such as the NEWS2. The clinicians who monitor James are suitably trained in their field and follow evidence-based interventions.

Patient experience: James' privacy and dignity are maintained throughout his stay. The nursing team treat him with dignity, empathy and compassion. At all stages in his care, James is informed, consent is gained and he is given opportunity to make decisions in his care.

James should receive the same care in all accident and emergency departments across the UK.

In the NHS and private healthcare providers, nursing leaders have a responsibility to monitor quality and challenge poor care, ensuring patients receive safe, effective and satisfactory care. A TNA can monitor quality and challenge poor care using the following:

1. *national standards*: use national standards, such as those developed by NICE or the CQC, to establish clear expectations for care delivery;
2. *local policies and procedures*: your organisation should develop local policies and procedures that align with national standards and provide clear guidance on how to deliver high-quality care. This can help nurses and other professionals to understand expectations for care delivery;

3. *developing a culture of improvement*: organisations and clinical leaders should foster a culture of continuous quality improvement in the team. This can include providing regular feedback to colleagues through supervision, identifying areas for improvement and promoting an environment where team members have access to training and development. As a TNA, you can support healthy cultures through role modelling;

4. *involving patients and families*: you should involve patients and their families in the care delivery process to ensure that their needs and preferences are met. You can achieve this by providing education and resources to patients and families, soliciting feedback on their experiences and involving them in decision-making processes;

5. *report incidents*: your organisation should encourage healthcare professionals to report incidents or near-misses to ensure that corrective action is taken, and that patient safety is improved;

6. *work collaboratively*: everyone should work collaboratively with other healthcare professionals, regulatory bodies and patient advocacy groups to improve care delivery and address poor care, ensuring that patient safety is the top priority and that appropriate action is taken to address poor care.

To ensure good-quality care, there must be examples of what good care looks like and clear standards to follow. In health, regulatory bodies such as the NMC provide the guidance we must follow to achieve a standard of quality that ensures services are clinically effective, safe and provide a good experience to those who use them. By following standards to monitor and challenge poor practice, you can help to ensure that patients receive high-quality care and that care providers are held accountable for the care they provide.

Below you will be introduced to examples of regulatory bodies, some of which you will have already come across in your journey to become a RNA. This chapter will cover their function in monitoring quality in care.

Professional regulators

You will be familiar with the regulatory body responsible for setting standards and guidance for NAs, the NMC. The NMC regulates individuals who want to practice as an RNA or nurse. First, the individual will need to complete a standard of training, such as the 2,300 hours of practice to complete before registration. In 2018 the NMC updated its standards for education and proficiencies which potential registrants need to achieve prior to practising as a registered nursing professional. You will know these as the NMC proficiencies you evidence in both your theory work and time in practice. The NMC also expects the higher education institutions to adhere to standards for the education, support and empowerment of trainee nurses and NAs (NMC, 2018a).

Once on the NMC register, registered nursing professionals adhere to *The Code: Professional Standards of Practice and Behaviour for Nurses, Midwives and Nursing Associates* (NMC, 2018a). If an individual were to harm a patient or bring the profession into disrepute, the NMC would arrange an investigation into the individual's practice and adherence to the NMC *Code* (2018a), applying sanctions on their ability to practise as a registered nursing professional. As a NA, you should expect your colleagues to conduct themselves in line with the NMC *Code*, as you would yourself. In Chater 8, your position as a role model will be explored, demonstrating the standards expected from you to influence the practice of others.

While the NMC regulates nursing, other healthcare professionals such as occupational therapists and physiotherapists have their own regulatory body, the Health and Care Professions Council (HCPC). Doctors are regulated through the General Medical Council (GMC) and have their own code of conduct and standards to ensure quality and good practice is maintained.

National Institute for Health and Care Excellence (NICE)

At this point in the book, you will be familiar with NICE guidelines and their importance to clinical practice across England and Wales. NICE was formed in 1997 as an agency to monitor, review and evaluate the clinical and cost effectiveness of health interventions in England and Wales. The organisation provides clinical guidelines and appraisals in new technology, using evidence-based reviews to recommend best practice to both health and social care. For NICE, evidence will inform guidance, and Quality Standards measure the effectiveness of a service in treating certain conditions.

The NICE Quality Standards are aspirational statements, derived from evidence-based guidance that health and social care providers should aim for to drive quality improvement (Baillie, 2014).

An example of a Quality Standard is *Patient Experience in Adult NHS Services: Quality Standard* [QS15] (2019). According to NICE, this standard can be achieved through the following statements.

1. People using adult NHS services are treated with empathy, dignity and respect.
2. People using adult NHS services understand the roles of healthcare professionals involved in their care and know how to contact them about their ongoing healthcare needs.
3. People using adult NHS services experience coordinated care with clear and accurate information exchange between relevant health and social care professionals.
4. People using adult NHS services experience care and treatment that is tailored to their needs and preferences.
5. People using adult NHS services have their preferences for sharing information with their family members and carers established, respected and reviewed throughout their care.
6. People using adult NHS services are supported in shared decision-making.

You will be familiar with these statements, as your education and experience as a TNA teaches you to treat people with empathy, dignity and respect and actively support their participation in care through person-centred practice. This is what quality care looks like; this is probably how you would want your family member to be treated while in hospital. To monitor the quality of care, and your practice area's adherence the Quality Standards, data and information must be gathered (please refer to Chapter 5). In this instance, NICE measures the standard through patient surveys and documentation in clinical notes, so if you have actively participated in shared decision-making, document it!

Activity 7.2   Research

As a TNA, you will not be in a position to identify quality standards linked to your practice area, but it might be helpful to know what they are, and how they influence quality improvement and expectations of care for your patient population.

Consider the following.

You have a placement with a care home for older people; what are the expectations for supporting mental well-being within the service user group? How would you measure that the service is providing quality care?

If you go to the NICE webpage (nice.org.uk) you can find the Quality Standards; use the search bar, or navigate the website to seek an answer.

An outline answer to this question is given at the end of the chapter.

Understanding the theory: Commissioning for Quality and Innovation (CQUIN)

To ensure quality care is adopted nationally, NHS England publishes annual Quality Indicator targets, CQUINs, which the NHS and NHS-funded healthcare providers must demonstrate compliance with.

CQUIN targets have both financial incentives and sanctions; your manager will be responsible for monitoring CQUIN targets within your clinical speciality. You may find your chosen practice area is targeted by Commissioning and Improvement – for example, an ongoing CQUIN for mental health services is to improve service users' physical health. To achieve this CQUIN, mental health teams must monitor physical health, include monitoring care plans, and encourage actions such as regular blood tests for high cholesterol.

CQUIN targets often reflect the current socio-political agenda or can be influenced by poor practice and never events in healthcare. A CQUIN target published for 2023–24 is 'CQUIN07: recording of and appropriate response to NEWS2 score for unplanned critical care admission'. The target is in response to the evidence from the Covid-19 pandemic that timely identification of deterioration in conditions through the NEWS2 monitoring can reduce the need for higher level of care (NHS England, 2023). In the UK, staffing pressure can have a significant impact on the quality of care, with essential vital observation monitoring being delayed or missed in critically unwell patients (Redfern et al., 2019).

As a TNA, awareness of current CQUIN targets in your practice areas will give you the opportunity to monitor the quality of care delivered, and role model commitment to contemporary health issues.

Care Quality Commission

If you have previous care experience, you might have prepared for and participated in a visit from the Care Quality Commission (CQC). The CQC is an independent regulator who makes sure all health and social care services provide safe, effective, compassionate and high-quality care. If a service falls below minimum expected standards, the CQC can work with the provider to create an action plan for improvement or take action against inadequate care (CQC, 2023).

During a CQC inspection a panel of inspectors will visit your team to observe, interview and audit. They may want to speak with the services users about their experience of the care received. The inspector may speak with you; they will ask you questions about your role and explore your knowledge on procedures to ensure safety and dignity are maintained, such as safeguarding (Brown and Hilson, 2014), which we will explore towards the end of this chapter.

The CQC have five questions they answer and publish on your team.

- Are services safe?
- Are services effective?
- Are services caring?
- Are services responsive to people's need?
- Are services well led?

They will evidence their publication using observation, interviews, data and documentation such as clinical notes, training records and equipment maintenance records – for example, fridge checks and cleaning rotas. As you progress in your career as an RNA, you will at some point be involved in a CQC inspection; you will take an active part in maintaining quality of care within your team and act as a role model of what 'good' looks like.

Healthcare Improvement Scotland

For England and the UK, the standards set by CQC and NICE are followed. If you live and work in Scotland, you will follow advice from Healthcare Improvement Scotland, which sets standards, guidelines and monitors health and social care services.

How do we monitor quality of care?

To monitor good-quality care, you need to familiarise yourself with standards expected; the standards are set you by the regulatory bodies, national guidelines and local policy, as we have covered so far. As a NA, you will delegate care to junior colleagues and coordinate the care of the unit for the day (please refer to Chapter 6, where delegation is covered in detail). You know what good care looks like; how do you monitor and review the care of your team members, or service as a whole? Consider this scenario: you are working with Joanna in a medical assessment unit. Joanna is a healthcare assistant and has been in post for six months; she often works with you to support a bay of patients.

You have delegated Joanna tasks, ensuring that her role and responsibilities are clearly defined and understood, and she understands her accountability for the care provided. You ensure Joanna has the competency, training and skills to safely provide the interventions and set communication expectations so Joanna can report changes in patient status or any concerns she has. To monitor Joanna's work, you can do the following:

- *monitor patient outcomes*: to ensure that care is being provided effectively. This can include reviewing patient records, observing Joanna while she interacts with patients and provides care, and speaking directly with patients and their families;
- *provide feedback and support*: you should provide regular feedback and support to those providing delegated care. You can monitor Joanna's work by offering clinical/ peer supervision on a regular basis. During supervision, you can give Joanna feedback on her practice, as discussed in Chapter 8. Clinical supervision promotes quality and safety of care by facilitating reflection on practice and personal and professional development (RCN, 2022b). In supervision you can recognise good performance, identify areas for improvement and provide resources to help your colleague improve their performance;
- *perform periodic evaluations*: as a nurse associate leader, you should perform periodic evaluations of the delegated care being provided to ensure that it meets established standards of care. You can do this though audits, peer review process, or patient, family and carer feedback.

In cases such as Mid-Staffordshire much of the poor quality in care was attributed to negative culture which did not support continual learning (Francis, 2013); supervision is recognised as a tool to promote a culture of reflection and learning (Tomlinson, 2015). Throughout your career, you will be in a position to support junior colleagues like Joanna; this provision is expected through the NMC *Standards of Practice*:

> Demonstrate an ability to support and motivate other members of the care team and interact confidently with them [and] demonstrate the ability to monitor and review the quality of care delivered, providing challenge and constructive feedback, when an aspect of care has been delegated to others.

> (NMC, 2018c, 4.2 and 4.6)

Activity 7.3   Critical thinking

Imagine that you are on placement in an acute mental health unit and shadowing support worker Jason to take the vital signs of 50-year-old Mo, who has reported feeling dizzy to the medical team. Mo's physical observations need to be recorded every four hours. Jason reports he is confident in taking the observations. You observe him use an electric blood pressure machine that records BP and pulse; he notes these down on the NEWS2 chart. Jason then takes Mo's temperature using a digital thermometer and notes this on the chart.

After Mo has left the clinic room, you help Jason clean the equipment. You look at the NEWS2 chart and see it is incomplete as the respiration, SpO2 and consciousness level is missing. You comment on these; Jason responds that he records the vital signs as he was taught to by a colleague when he started on the ward.

What do you think the risks are and what action would you take?

Answers will be at the end of this chapter.

The role of patient and carer feedback in monitoring quality

Patient and carer feedback can be a powerful tool to monitor and review the quality of care we provide. In NHS services patients are encouraged to participate in feedback through surveys and questionnaires. If you have been working in a large hospital you may have seen patient satisfaction survey points in high-traffic areas such as reception, waiting areas or cafeterias. Patient feedback is valuable to service improvement, quality and safety. A common test used is the Friends and Family Test, launched in 2013 to provide an accessible method for the public to give feedback on services (NHS England, 2020).

Another novel resource to gain feedback from the public is through Care Opinion (www.careopinion.org.uk), a website that enables people who have used a service to tell their story of experiences in care. By sharing their stories, organisations can make improvements to healthcare delivery (Care Opinion, 2022).

During your career, you will certainly be faced with a situation where you need to support a patient or their family member to make a complaint. The NHS must ensure that complaints are acknowledged, investigated and responded to (Nandasoma, 2019); therefore, as a registered professional you will take an active role in enabling this process to happen. Each NHS trust will have its own complaints procedure and policy for you to follow. To manage complaints, you need to demonstrate your communication skills, including active listening, empathy and compassion (Gage, 2016). Most complaints may be managed at service level, avoiding escalation; however, all complaints should provide opportunity for learning and influence service improvement.

Audit

In Chapter 5 we explored how data and information impacts the way we practise nursing and its role in patient safety. We previously introduced the concept of data collection for audit in Chapter 5, using the NICE (2015) *Pressure Ulcers: Quality Standard* [QS89], which we will revisit in this chapter. While an audit can be undertaken for a variety of reasons, you may find it useful to monitor a team's performance against standards and frameworks, such as the NICE Quality Standards. The role of audit can be undertaken by anyone in your team, but it is an essential skill to meet within the

Healthcare Leadership Model (NHS Leadership Academy, 2023). According to NICE (2002, p. 69), 'Clinical audit is a quality improvement process that seeks to improve patient care and outcomes through systematic review of care against explicit criteria and the implementation of change.'

There is often confusion between a clinical audit, service evaluation and research projects. A *clinical audit* is a process to determine if a service is meeting established and defined standards of practice. You will use clinical audit to monitor quality of an aspect of care and often a clinical audit can lead to service improvement projects. A service evaluation measures the effectiveness of a service and seeks to demonstrate the service achieves its purpose. Finally, a research project is usually conducted to further our knowledge on a subject or create new theory.

Understanding the theory: the Clinical Audit Cycle (Benjamin, 2008)

To ensure the success of our audit and avoid wasting clinicians' time, a systematic process is recommended (NICE, 2002). Benjamin's Audit Cycle (2008) outlines the necessary steps for achieving changes in practice.

- Stage 1: Preparing for audit
- Stage 2: Selecting criteria for audit review
- Stage 3: Measuring level of performance
- Stage 4: Making improvements
- Stage 5: Sustaining improvements

Audits can be used to assess resource utilisation, care processes and outcomes, such as whether patients on an acute mental health unit have a physical healthcare plan, or what the waiting time for a particular therapy is. Audits are usually conducted retrospectively, using data from clinical notes, care plans and documentation. As we discussed in Chapter 5, high-quality data and documentation are essential for meaningful audit results.

For further reading on Benjamin's Clinical Audit Cycle, please refer to the additional reading list at the end of this chapter.

To illustrate a clinical audit cycle in practice, let's imagine you are on placement in a medical assessment unit (MAU), as we saw in Chapter 5. Due to an increase in hospital-acquired pressure ulcers in the regional area, your unit manager has proposed an audit to monitor the quality of care within the MAU; you have volunteered to participate in the audit team to achieve proficiency in 5.2 'participate in data collection to support audit activity, and contribute to the implementation of quality improvement strategies', as outlined by the NMC (2018c).

To begin the audit, you need to select the topic of investigation. Fortunately, the prevention pressure ulcers is a familiar topic to quality improvement and audit cycles (Kottner et al., 2018). To pick your topic, you will need to access evidence-based standards and framework. In audit, you are asking 'are we doing the right thing the right way?' (Benjamin, 2008). For pressure ulcers, you can access the NICE guidelines and Quality Standards on the topic, or if you are in Scotland the *Prevention and Management of Pressure Ulcers* (HIS, 2020). Let us take NICE (2015) Quality Standards for pressure ulcers as an example. These should demonstrate evidence-based interventions that prevent skin deterioration and evidence what quality care should look like.

The next stage is collecting the data for your audit. Deciding what data to collect for a complex topic such as pressure ulcers can be confusing, so you may want to seek advice from your local audit or quality improvement team. There may be an audit tool provided by NICE, such as the NICE (2014) clinical audit tool, for pressure ulcer prevention. Using this tool, you will select a sample of patients who have received care and review their clinical records to collect the data needed.

From the data you have collected, you can identify areas of good performance – such as that 90 per cent of patients receive a pressure ulcer assessment within six hours of admission – as well as areas where performance is inadequate or not reported. The information you get from your audit can support service improvement projects and staff development.

Another audit you may be familiar with is the hand hygiene audit. Hand hygiene and infection control are fundamental aspects of nursing practice and good hand washing technique reduces the risk of hospital-acquired infections. Regular hand hygiene audits are recommended to ensure adherence to hand hygiene guidelines (Loveday et al., 2014).

To conduct a hand hygiene audit, you may use an audit box with a UV light and stop members of the multidisciplinary team (MDT) working in your unit. You will check if they are compliant with the dress code, such as being bare below the elbows, wearing minimal jewellery and having short, clean nails. The member of staff will then wash a UV cream from their hands using handwashing technique and be inspected under the UV light. The data from the audit should be recorded and displayed in line with the NICE guidelines on *Healthcare-associated Infections: Prevention and Control* (NICE, 2012). This is a simple yet effective audit that promotes quality and safety of care, and it is a leadership role that a TNA or RNA can take on a local level.

Challenging poor care and when to escalate

So far in this chapter you have explored what quality of care is, who sets the standards for care quality and how we monitor the standards are met within our practice area. Unfortunately, poor practice is not uncommon in the UK, and you may witness care which does not meet standards, or is neglectful and, on rare occasions, abusive.

Case study: Toxic cultures

In October 2022 the BBC broadcast their investigation into poor care at Edenfield Mental Health Centre in Greater Manchester. Edenfield is a medium-secure mental health service, where vulnerable people with complex mental health conditions are sectioned and detained under the Mental Health Act (1983). The hospital provides care for both male and female service users, who have an average admission of two years.

The investigation was prompted after allegations of misconduct and whistle-blowing from staff members went largely ignored. The hospital had recently received a 'Good' rating from its recent CQC inspection. During the investigation from the BBC, a 'toxic culture of abuse' was uncovered, including bullying, sexualised behaviour towards patients, falsified observation records and unprofessional behaviour from a small group of staff (*Panorama*, 2022). A full independent inquiry into the failing and abuse at Edenfield is currently in progress (Mind, 2023). The BBC investigation is available to watch on BBC iPlayer, a recommendation if you are planning to practice in mental health services.

Although the full inquiry into Edenfield is underway, there are similarities from pre-existing investigations of poor care in both Mid-Staffordshire and Winterbourne View of toxic cultures which enabled abuse and poor-quality care to develop (DoH, 2012; Francis, 2013). A workplace culture can be defined as the character and personality of an organisation (Skills for Care, 2018) which has shared values and morals within a team. A positive culture in healthcare encourages inclusion, fairness, support and people put at the heart of the service (Skills for Care, 2018). Poor workplace cultures increase the risk of harm to service users and are more likely to develop in long-term care facilities with weak leadership, poor training and development for staff and lack of communication and opportunity to speak up (CQC, 2022).

The consequence of a toxic culture can lead to financial loss, staff bullying, reduced quality of care and, in severe cases, abusive behaviour towards vulnerable people receiving care. It is recognised that leadership can improve care and reduce the risk of toxic workplace cultures developing. As a TNA, you should use your leadership, role modelling and teamwork skills to contribute to positive cultures within your work environment, challenging negative cultures and raising concerns.

What does poor care look like?

While a negative culture can have devastating impact on the quality of care, morale of staff and patient satisfaction, these environments develop over time and creep into organisations and teams. Maintaining safe work environment is everyone's responsibility and, as a TNA, you can role model good care and monitor the effectiveness of your team. However, first it is important to understand what poor-quality care looks like. A good measure for quality of care is through the lens of the CQC.

Earlier in the chapter, we explored the role of a CQC inspection to maintain quality of care through the *five key questions*: are services safe, effective, caring, responsive and well led? Let's imagine an example in which services might not meet the minimum standard of quality required.

Safe – A safe service has adequate staff on duty, who have the right skills, education and knowledge to support patients. Currently, the NHS, health and social care are experiencing a staffing crisis. Understaffing may feel like an inevitability and just 'how it's done', but it has significant impacts on the quality of care and safety of patients. A systematic review by Recio-Saucedo et al. (2018) highlighted moderate evidence that low staffing numbers leads to 'missed care' such as incomplete nursing jobs; think back to vital observations being missed or omitted from earlier in this chapter.

Every ward will have an agreed staffing ratio by which it can protect the safety and care standards. This is decided based on number of patients, acuity and complexity of the patient group using the ward. If you are regularly working in a team, you may want to discuss the safer staffing level of the ward with a senior nurse or manager. It feels inevitable that there will be days we work with a 'skeleton staff', the minimum number to keep the ward safe, but are you aware when your ward is below the agreed staffing?

According to safer staffing initiative (National Quality Board, 2013) all wards must have the right number of suitably trained staff who are in the right place at the right time. This might look like a suitable number of registered nurses, male and female members of the nursing team, with staff suitably trained to work within emergencies, such as a cardiac arrest. As a TNA, what can you do if your team do not have suitable staffing? If there is the option, you may need to approach a close ward for cover or a staff member swap to ensure correct numbers and skills mix or approach your manager to request additional staffing be employed through staff bank or agency. It is important to document that staffing has fallen below expected standard; we will cover the reasons why towards the end of the chapter.

If you need to read more to imagine what poor care looks like, use your web browser to search for recent healthcare scandals across England: the Francis Report (Francis, 2013), Winterbourne View (DoH, 2012) or BBC documentaries that are listed in the further reading section.

Incident reporting, safeguarding and whistle-blowing

As a TNA, you may have to report an incident, near-miss or raise a concern of practice. For the final section of the chapter, we will explore what you can do if you are concerned about poor practice. It is important to remember each organisation will have their own policy for incident reporting, safeguarding and raising concerns; you should familiarise yourself with these in your induction period.

You may have come across incident reporting by this point in your journey to become a registrant; however, do you understand why you create incident reports, what is done with the information and how clear incident reporting contributes to patient safety? Incident reporting involves documenting any unplanned event that could have or has caused harm to a patient, staff member, or visitor, including near-misses and adverse events. These events can include medication errors, falls, pressure ulcers, misidentification of patients and equipment failure. Incident reporting aims to identify the root causes of incidents, prevent future occurrences and improve patient safety (NHS England, 2015).

At a local level, the information from incident reporting can be used to solve clinical issues – for example, if a high incidence of falls is noticed within a ward, is there a solution within the environment? Data collected through your local incident reporting system are analysed through national reporting systems, allowing for large volumes of data to contribute towards national agenda, medication safety and policy (NHS Improvement, 2019) – a good incentive to remember your responsibility in clear reporting and documentation, as we outlined in Chapter 5.

To promote patient safety and a culture of reporting, it is essential that incident reporting remains blame free. Incident reporting is not about finding a person to blame when care goes wrong, but supporting change and learning from error.

Over your training and career, there is a possibility you will encounter care that has fallen below standard and puts patients, public and staff at risk from harm. In these instances, you may have to speak out and raise concerns to protect well-being, health and human rights. Everyone has a responsibility to ensure safeguarding policy is followed; however, as a TNA, you have a duty to: 'Act without delay if you believe that there is a risk to patient safety or public protection' (NMC, 2018a, p. 17). Your organisation will have a local policy for reporting safeguarding and a designated individual to discuss concerns you have. You can raise concerns through the appropriate channels in your workplace or go directly to the NMC or CQC. If you are currently a student and want to raise a concern over something you have witnessed in practice or you have seen in placement, the higher education institution will have its own reporting process, so talk to your personal tutor or course lead.

Stages of raising concerns

The NMC guidance for raising concerns (NMC, 2019a) guides all registrants and students on the appropriate steps to take when concerned about the safety and well-being of people in their care. The NMC (2019a) states that all nursing professionals have a duty of care to speak up and report their concerns if the safety of patients is compromised. You have a duty of care to protect the public and yourself, to not be given excessive workload and practise out of your skill and competency (RCN, 2023). If you are in the position where you have a concern, you should follow the appropriate guidance from your local trust policy and seek advice from your union if outside support as needed. As a leader, you should extend this support to junior colleagues, ensuring they are supported to raise concerns without judgement or repercussion.

Throughout raising a concern, you need to take immediate action if there is imminent risk of harm; this will be taken to an appropriate person or authority. You may have a *speak up guardian* (National Guardian's Office, 2021) allocated in your organisation who you can contact if you do not feel you are able to speak to a line manager. Where you need to raise a concern, you will still need to consider your patient confidentiality. If you have a concern, keep a record of any actions you take, or any events you have witnessed.

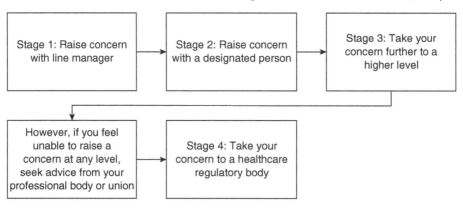

Figure 7.1 Raising a concern

Source: Adapted from NMC (2019a).

Chapter summary

Over this chapter we have explored the meaning of quality in care and how we monitor and challenge poor care in practice. Regulatory bodies and national guidelines will set out standards for all healthcare professionals to follow to deliver care that is safe, clinically effective and give patients, families and carers good experience of care.

You can monitor quality care though peer supervision, patient and public feedback and clinical audit. Participating in these will be part of your role as an RNA and nurse leader. Monitoring care and documentation leads to improved services and patient safety. When standards fall below expectation, staff morale is low and training and development opportunities are not available, a negative culture can develop within a team or organisation. As a nurse leader, you can promote positive culture through role modelling and supervision.

To report poor care, you can approach your line manager or speak up guardian. As a registrant under the NMC you have a duty of care to document and report incidents and concerns. This should not be about blame, but opportunity for learning from error and maintaining patient safety.

Activities: brief outline answers

Activity 7.2

The guidance you need will be under 'Mental health and wellbeing'; there is Quality Standard *Mental Wellbeing of Older People in Care Homes: Quality Standard* [QS50] (NICE, 2013). The quality standard covers people over the age of 65 receiving care in a care home environment, which is suitable advice for your placement in the care home.

There are six statements:

- Quality Statement 1: Participation in meaningful activity
- Quality Statement 2: Personal identity
- Quality Statement 3: Recognition of mental health conditions
- Quality Statement 4: Recognition of sensory impairment
- Quality Statement 5: Recognition of physical problems
- Quality Statement 6: Access to healthcare services

These are aspirational statements of achieving quality care for the mental well-being of care home residents. To achieve these statements, you will ensure that all residents have these needs addressed in their care plan and documented in clinical notes. To measure the effectiveness of the care given, you may consider patient surveys or audit.

Activity 7.3

Vital signs are integral to monitoring the condition of patients. Respiration rate and SpO2 may be the first sign of deterioration, therefore missing the recording of these can put Mo in danger of a sudden deterioration (Elliott, 2021).

As a TNA, you might have identified an oversight of the training process on the ward, and it would be part of your role to investigate further. Jason may have been advised wrong by a well-meaning member of staff, or perhaps the team are unaware of the evidence-base behind the NEWS2 chart. After discussion with your practice supervisor, you could audit the NEWS2 charts to provide evidence for your concern; if a problem is identified, as a TNA, you could deliver a teaching session for the staff.

Further reading

Francis, R. (2013) *Report of the Mid Staffordshire NHS Foundation Trust Public Inquiry.* London: HMSO.

The Francis Report (2013) is an independent report on the failings of Mid-Staffordshire NHS Trust. You may have encountered this report within your study.

Department of Health (2012) *Transforming Care: A National Response to Winterbourne View Hospital.* London: DoH.

An independent review into the failings of a learning disability provider.

NICE (2013) *Mental Wellbeing of Older People in Care Homes: Quality Standard* [QS50]. London: NICE. Available at: www.nice.org.uk/guidance/qs50

This is an example of a NICE Quality Standard to familiarise yourself with. Especially relevant for a placement in a care home.

Panorama (2022) Undercover hospital: patients at risk. BBC. Available at: www.bbc.co.uk/iplayer/episode/m001ckxr/panorama-undercover-hospital-patients-at-risk

A documentary looking into poor care in a mental health inpatient unit.

Benjamin, A. (2008) Audit: how to do it in practice. *BMJ*, 336(7655): 1241–1245.

An article in the *BMJ*, which explains the audit process in healthcare.

Useful websites

www.cqc.org.uk/

Care Quality Commission website which has some useful information regarding CQC inspections and quality care standards.

www.nmc.org.uk/globalassets/blocks/media-block/raising-concerns-v2.pdf

NMC guidance for raising concerns from practice.

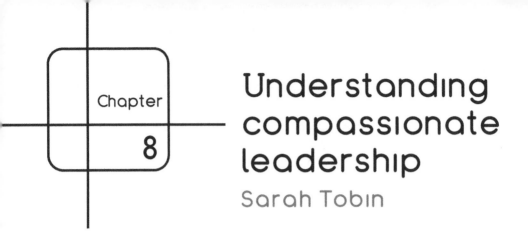

Chapter 8

Understanding compassionate leadership

Sarah Tobin

Chapter aims

After reading this chapter you will be able to:

- describe and discuss the importance of compassionate leadership and cultures and ways in which this can be achieved;

- understand the definition and context of compassion and how this relates to leadership in nursing;
- be aware of the rationale for prioritising the skill of compassion and the impact this has on staff well-being, patient care and safety;
- appreciate the importance of role modelling, providing feedback and exercising duty of candour;
- link reflective practice and self-awareness to compassionate leadership and self-compassion.

Introduction

This chapter will explore the importance of compassion and the way that using the 'skill' of compassion can impact how effective you are as a leader. The subject and study of compassion is popular in healthcare, with a significant amount of research, opinion and literature devoted to this over recent years. It is important to be clear about what is meant by the word *compassion* so that discussions can be informed and relevant; a definition will be presented.

According to the Department of Health and Social Care (2021, Principle 3) 'Respect, dignity, compassion and care should be at the core of how patients and staff are treated not only because that is the right thing to do but because patient safety, experience and outcomes are all improved when staff are valued, empowered and supported.' This indicates that when practising as a nurse, and especially when acting in a leadership role, this must be done with compassion. This requirement is not simply because it is a nice thing to do – it has significant clinical impact as research has found that patients who are treated by compassionate staff do better. Compassion also has implications for staff and the wider team: when a culture is compassionate staff are less likely to leave. So, this chapter will also include a section exploring how compassionate leadership creates a compassionate culture.

In recognition of the impact of compassionate practice, the word *compassion* now features much more frequently in healthcare policy and in protocols and guidelines. In the *Standards of Proficiency* (NMC, 2018c), Platform 1, which relates to being an accountable professional, says that you are expected to provide nursing care that is 'person-centred, safe and compassionate'. Platform 3 states that you will provide 'compassionate, safe and effective care' and Annex A suggests that sensitive and compassionate communication is 'central' to how you will carry out your role. One way to enhance your compassion skills or to share those that you have is by following or being a compassionate role model; this chapter includes a discussion about how it is possible to role model compassionate practice and leadership.

Allied to this are the skills of providing feedback to those you work with and the need to be open and honest and how this can be achieved without compromising a compassionate focus. In the final section, this chapter will describe the importance of reflection and self-awareness as a way of enhancing your ability to practice compassionately and to acknowledge the importance of self-compassion.

So - what is compassion?

Think back to Tina's case study in Chapter 4 relating the experience of a nurse on night duty who made a drug error. Such a mistake is a serious issue; remember, drug errors result in significant harm and cost. So, those who act as managers and who are accountable for supervising and leading colleagues are neither expected nor permitted to simply ignore a staff member who makes a drug error. When a leader has no choice in a course of action – such as a formal disciplinary process, for instance – it is important that this process is followed and followed according to agreed and accepted protocols and policies. However, where managers and leaders do have choice is in how they work with the protocols and policies and how they apply them. They can choose how the process can best be used to, in the case in the scenario, protect and promote patient safety, but also how this can be achieved as effectively and positively for the staff members involved. In the scenario the correct process may well have been followed (see below) but, at the end of that process, the nurse involved resigned and her colleagues were left feeling that they might not report errors in future – neither outcome beneficial to patient safety. The question is, therefore, could the process have been followed in a way that resulted in a better, safer outcome for all concerned?

Activity 8.1   Reflection

Please re-read the case study given in Chapter 4, pp. 63, relating to Tina. As mentioned, this case was based on a real nurse and her experience. In that case the nurse was subsequently suspended from administering drugs while awaiting the outcome of a disciplinary process. This lasted over six weeks and resulted in a formal warning and a compulsory training update for medicines management. The nurse reported that she felt humiliated as she had to ask others to cover her drug rounds and explain why; she felt angry at how she had been treated. It was the 'worst six weeks of her career' and shortly after this she resigned. Other nurses on the ward were reported as saying that witnessing this process meant that they would be reluctant to report any drug errors in future.

What are your immediate feelings about the impact on the nurse involved?

- Do you think the relevant disciplinary policy was applied appropriately?
- Do you think the policy was applied compassionately?
- Do you believe that a policy designed to support disciplinary measures can or should be considered with compassion in mind?
- Do you think the outcome was inevitable and provided overall benefit to patient care?

Whatever your thoughts and ideas are, make a note, consider how you felt when reading the scenario: what would you have said to the nurse concerned if you were her colleague?

As this is a reflective exercise no outline answer is provided at the end of the chapter.

It would be difficult to find many people who would argue that compassion should not be at the heart of healthcare practice. However, there are always different perspectives and these will be explored later in the chapter. For now, we need to have a common understanding; if a discussion is called for and the subject is 'four-legged things' and one person is talking about a chair and someone else is talking about a hippopotamus you can appreciate why confusion can arise! Good leadership, as with meaningful discussion, relies on creating a common understanding.

Understanding what is meant by the term *compassion* is complicated by the interchangeability of terms such as *empathy, sympathy, caring, altruism, kindness* and so on. Sinclair et al. (2017) explored the meanings of these terms. They identified that a clear definition is important to help support research which will then guide clinical practice.

Understanding the theory: defining compassion

Strauss et al. (2016, p. 15) suggest that without an agreed definition it is not possible to 'study compassion, measure compassion or evaluate whether interventions designed to enhance compassion are effective'.

Providing a definition is challenging as, while dictionary entries are technically correct, they are not subtle nor comprehensive enough to explain the quality that is expected of healthcare workers. Linguistically, the term *compassion* is derived from the Latin root 'com', which means 'together with' and 'pati', which is 'to bear or suffer'. This definition – in essence to suffer with – is equally contentious in healthcare professions, where the body of evidence to support the increasing level of *burnout* and *compassion fatigue* is overwhelming. It is important that we care for and about our patients, but I think we can all see the problems that would develop if we suffered alongside them.

Some healthcare professionals may even argue that there is a need to be more dispassionate to enable them to carry out their role. This was an idea explored in the work of Anna Smajdor (2013), who suggested it can be damaging for healthcare professionals to feel too much compassion – because they may become deeply distressed by some of the things they see and do. They are at risk of suffering burnout, fatigue, becoming de-sensitised and damaged.

A recent review by Malenfant et al. (2022) highlights the fact that there is ongoing research and discussion about the nature of compassion so it is clear that the debate about the subject continues. This study did make an important point – that compassion is different from empathy (perhaps the most used alternative word). The difference between the two concepts relates to *action*: empathy compels us to care about someone, but compassion compels us to do something about their suffering.

For the purpose of this chapter, it is important that we can agree a common understanding, so we will need a definition. Gilbert (2017) suggests that compassion is 'a sensitivity to suffering in self and others with a commitment to try to alleviate and prevent it'. We can accept that this concise definition is based on sound research and is as well-evidenced as any other. Most importantly, we now need to address how compassion can be 'used' as a skill to enhance leadership, followership and, therefore, patient care.

Case study: Mr and Mrs J

The following is a real case study taken from the *Care and Compassion? Report of the Health Service Ombudsman on Ten Investigations into NHS Care of Older People* (PHSO, 2010, pp. 11–12). It perhaps demonstrates clearly why compassion is a very necessary component of caring for people.

Mrs J was 82 years old. She had Alzheimer's disease and lived in a nursing home. Her husband visited her daily and they enjoyed each other's company. Mr J told us 'She had been like that for nine years. And I was happy being with her'. One evening, Mr J arrived at the home and found that his wife had breathing difficulties. An ambulance was called and Mrs J was taken to Ealing Hospital NHS Trust at about 10.30pm, accompanied by her husband. She was admitted to A&E and assessed on arrival by a Senior House Officer who asked Mr J to wait in a waiting room.

Mrs J was very ill. She was taken to the resuscitation area but was moved later when two patients arrived who required emergency treatment. Mrs J was then seen by a Specialist Registrar as she was vomiting and had become unresponsive. It was decided not to resuscitate her. She died shortly after 1.00am. At around 1.40am the nursing staff telephoned the nursing home and were told that Mr J had accompanied his wife to hospital. The Senior House Officer found him in the waiting room and informed him that his wife had died.

In the three hours or so that Mr J had been in the waiting room, nobody spoke to him or told him what was happening to his wife. As a result, he came to believe that her care had been inadequate. He thought that he had been deliberately separated from her because hospital staff had decided to stop treating her. 'They let her slip away under the cloak of "quality of life" without stopping to think of any other involved party.' He felt the hospital had denied them the chance to be together in the last moments of Mrs J's life and he did not know what had happened to her.

The Ombudsman's investigation found that the decision not to resuscitate Mrs J was correct but that there had been a significant failing in communication as it should have been *'crucial that Mr J was involved in the decision-making and the move to compassionate and supportive care in his wife's last moments. Mrs J was denied the right to a dignified death with her husband by her side'*. The failing was not because of a lack of clinical expertise but because of a lack of care and compassion.

Compassionate leadership creates compassionate cultures

The National Health Service is one of the largest single employers on the planet. The people who provide care for patients are the greatest determinant of the effectiveness of that care. Not the only determinant, obviously physical resources play a part, but it is obvious that an effective workforce will, in turn, provide effective care.

It is clear that compassionate care results in better outcomes for patients and for staff but while this seems simple it can be a real challenge to ensure that this happens. If a member of staff does not feel they are being shown compassion, then evidence suggests that they will find it harder to provide compassionate care to patients or behave compassionately towards fellow employees. A 'leader' has an obligation to ensure that staff are treated compassionately, and this requires that the culture or approach of the organisation that they work in is based on an intent to be compassionate.

The Courage of Compassion (West et al., 2020) highlights the need to provide compassionate leadership and a compassionate culture in which to work. They suggest three ways this might be achieved.

1. *Autonomy*: staff need to feel that they have some control over their working life and that they can work in a way that reflects their values.
2. *Belonging*: staff need to be connected, to feel cared for and to be able to care for others around them at work, they need to feel valued respected and supported.
3. *Contribution*: people need to feel that they are effective in what they do and that they deliver valued outcomes.

Activity 8.2   Critical thinking

Thinking about these three ways to achieve a compassionate culture – known as the ABC framework – imagine that you are working on a shift with colleagues; there are several team members whom you are supervising. What could you do to try and ensure that you lead these colleagues in a way that reflects the three requirements described above?

If it helps, you can read *The Courage of Compassion* report (West et al., 2020) on the King's Fund website, where you will find recommendations including practical steps that can be taken.

An outline answer is provided at the end of this chapter.

West et al. (2020) also acknowledged the impact of significant levels of vacant posts in the nursing and midwifery workforce. Despite the huge numbers of staff who work in the NHS, the Nuffield Trust (2022) suggest that one in thirteen posts are currently vacant. Even more concerning is that, according to the latest *NHS Staff Survey* (NHS, 2021), nearly a third of staff reported that they often thought about leaving their job and nearly half reported feeling unwell because of work-related stress. While the Covid-19 pandemic, which began in 2020, has undoubtedly had an impact, the 2018 *Staff Survey* (NHS, 2018) reported that a very similar percentage of staff were considering leaving and that nearly 40 per cent felt unwell because of workplace stress. With significant vacancies adding to these pressures, it would appear that the survey respondents in 2018 may well have acted on their wish to leave. It is vital therefore that all steps are taken to encourage people to stay in the workforce, and avoid the cycle of burnout and staff dissatisfaction.

In 2018, burnout was listed as an actual illness by the World Health Organization (WHO) and described as: 'a syndrome resulting from chronic work stress' and that it features 'emotional exhaustion, depersonalization (cynicism, loss of idealism, withdrawal), and feeling ineffective' (WHO, 2019). The RCN (2022c) called it *compassion fatigue*, and suggested that when compassion exists in a clinical team (for patients and for each other) that team will not only be more effective, but patient safety and satisfaction will also be higher. West (2021) also highlights the relationship between the absence of compassionate cultures and the increase in levels of burnout. As an 'antidote' he cites a study which demonstrated that compassion was one of the most potent activators of brain circuits associated with happiness. Staff who can be compassionate and who are treated with compassion are happy staff!

As a matter of concern, cultures that lack compassion are also more likely to discriminate against their workforce. The 2021 *NHS Staff Survey* reported that only just over half of all respondents felt that their organisation provided equal opportunities and this figure was significantly less among people from ethnic minority backgrounds. This is echoed by the Nuffield Trust (2022), which highlights that while approximately 25 per cent of NHS staff are from an ethnic minority background (much higher than the 13 per cent of all working-age adults in the UK), this group of staff are under-represented in Agenda for Change Band 6 roles and even more so at Band 8. Both the NHS and the social care sector employ significantly more women than men – in fact, with over a million, the NHS is possibly the largest employer of women in the world! Along with race and disability, gender is one of the characteristics where increasing discrimination is reported. As a significant employer of people from ethnic minority backgrounds and of women it is imperative that the NHS ensures fairness, inclusion and lack of discrimination.

As described earlier in this book, leadership is not a 'role' – it is an aspect of everyone's practice and certainly an expectation of nursing associates (NAs). Being compassionate as a leader has been shown to help keep staff from leaving, help staff to be happier and more fulfilled in their work and increase the level of inclusion and opportunity for valuing diversity in all forms.

Activity 8.3   Critical thinking

This chapter has suggested that, as NAs, if you lead and practise with compassion then patients will have a better clinical outcome. Think about this and list the reasons why you think that this might be the case – what is it about compassionate care that results in better patient outcomes?

To help your thoughts and ideas – find and watch the fifteen-minute YouTube video of a TED talk given by Dr Stephen Trzeciak, who is an intensive care doctor and researcher in the USA.

A model answer is included at the end of this chapter.

Role modelling compassionate leadership practice - to yourself and others

So – this chapter has described and defined compassion, discussed the impact and rationale for being compassionate but ... how can we be compassionate? How do we *do it*?

First, it is important to acknowledge that people are innately compassionate – the definition of a person without compassion is a psychopath! I think that you will have worked with some people who demonstrated greater levels of compassion than others, but I think it is unlikely that you have worked with someone who is a psychopath. So, perhaps it is therefore important to think about how we can encourage people to maximise their compassion potential, to use the resources they already have. One way that this can happen is to look for compassionate role models and to be one yourself.

Think about the job that nurses do: how often have you worked with a colleague in a leadership role who regularly does not take their breaks or who stays significantly past the end of their shift? This may seem like the actions of a committed and conscientious nurse but how sustainable is this? What happens if this behaviour not only becomes the norm but also the expected level of behaviour in the team? To provide compassionate leadership a leader must first practise and role model self-compassion. If a person does not acknowledge their own needs and challenges, then they may struggle to recognise or understand those of their colleagues. This includes being aware of your own vulnerability, needs and human failings and accepting that these will also be present in your colleagues.

Language is a very important way of demonstrating compassionate intent but also of providing a role model for your colleagues to follow – words can become actions and can determine the culture of a shift and even an entire working environment.

Case study: Casey

Casey is a nineteen-year-old girl who frequently attends the emergency department (ED). She left school at sixteen and has not been in either education or employment since then. Casey has lived at several different addresses in the three years since she left the family home; these include 'sofa-surfing' with friends, a period cohabiting with a boyfriend and a short period where she was homeless.

Casey has previously attended ED due to an overdose of prescribed antidepressants, because of injuries that were unexplained but possibly as a result of domestic abuse and because of various attempts to harm herself. On several occasions Casey has been removed from the ED by security staff due to her abusive and violent behaviour.

In the middle of a busy shift Casey attends the department; an experienced NA hears a commotion in the waiting room and, on investigation, finds Casey shouting at the

(Continued)

(Continued)

reception staff, accusing them of being rude to her and 'rolling their eyes'. Casey has obvious injuries to her arms and these are oozing blood.

The NA addresses Casey by her name, says 'Hello' and tells her he will find a private space to assess her wounds. Telling her that he is sorry to see Casey here today but that he will do his best to help her, the NA leads Casey to a cubicle. Casey begins to cry and apologises for shouting and asks if she could please have a cup of tea as she hasn't eaten for several days and is feeling faint.

Activity 8.4   Reflection

Do you feel sorry for Casey or can you understand why some staff may have 'rolled their eyes'? Why do you think Casey starts to cry?

What do you think will be the benefit to Casey, to the NA and to the ED because of the way the NA approached Casey?

A suggested answer is included at the end of the chapter.

There is a saying, 'If you always do what you've always done, you'll always get what you always got'! A neat way of recognising that we need to change what we do if we want a different outcome. A study as long ago as 1995 by Redelmeier et al. recognised this and examined whether treating patients just like Casey with compassion could change anything. The study randomised repeat ED attenders who were homeless to either standard care or to standard care plus compassionate input from volunteers. The results indicated a drop in the number of return visits by those patients who were treated with compassion by about 30 per cent. Compassion is a powerful tool, words matter and patient care and experience can be improved by the simple application of kindness. A reduction of repeat visits to the ED is also a significant cost saving, so compassionate care is also expedient and sustainable.

Activity 8.5   Reflection

Consider the following:

a) You are heading in to work, your day has started well and you are feeling posi-tive, happy and are looking forward to the day ahead. You enter the ward and the nurse who has been in charge on the night shift greets you with, 'You don't want to be here, it has been chaos, awful – everything has gone wrong and we're running late. It's hell – thank goodness I can hand over – I can't wait to get out of here!'

Or:

b) You are heading in to work, your day has started well and you are feeling positive, happy and are looking forward to the day ahead. You enter the ward and the nurse who has been in charge on the night shift greets you with, 'I'm pleased to see you, we've had a busy night with some challenges and I'm afraid that some things have been left but we've kept everyone safe and did the best we could. I'd like to finish off and go home as soon as I can, so let me hand over what has happened and what is left to do.'

It really can be as simple as this – imagine how you would feel if your day started as described above. How would you feel in each scenario, how would it affect your mood, your level of enthusiasm and your approach to the rest of the day?

As this is a reflective exercise no model answer has been provided.

We have a choice: in the activity above you can be the first nurse or you can demonstrate consideration, understanding and leadership and be the second nurse. Importantly, evidence shows that rudeness or snappiness towards colleagues has a significant negative impact not only on their subsequent performance but also that of any team members who witness the event. The King's Fund (2022) highlights the 'compelling link between compassion in leadership and staff wellbeing, team performance, and better outcomes for patients and service users. The NHS People Plan even recognises compassion as a national priority.'

Providing feedback: a skill that needs practice

Another way a leader can role model compassion is in the way that they provide feedback to their colleagues. This chapter has already discussed the challenges that exist when a leader needs to manage disciplinary procedures and how this can be done with a compassionate focus, but what about everyday feedback? Providing feedback is essential to good, effective team-working but can be a daunting concept and, as a result, is an element of leadership that some people may avoid. However, providing feedback is an innately compassionate act and not to do so is to the detriment of both the individual and the team.

Michael West (2021) writes about this in his book on compassionate leadership, but the essence of his ideas include that we need to listen to each other, identify what problems exist and may be impacting on a person's behaviour, demonstrate understanding of people's challenges, share that learning and jointly devise and agree any solutions. Compassionate feedback is not a *one off* activity but part of the culture of a workplace – once objectives are agreed they need to be monitored and, crucially, supported.

The NHS has created a toolkit (NHS England, 2022a) to promote their Civility and Respect Framework and part of this toolkit suggests ways to bring about changes in behaviour that do not make a person feel blamed or punished. One of the key messages is that feedback needs to be given and that the earlier an issue is identified the more likelihood that simple measures can be adopted to prevent a problem escalating. The toolkit suggests that a compassionate approach is highlighted by a respectful and supportive interaction, they call it an 'informal cup of coffee intervention'. The key point is that it is kinder to address concerns as soon as they arise and that by doing so it is often possible to prevent problems from escalating. You may have heard colleagues say 'I wish someone had told me' when problems have arisen and this is probably how you would want to be treated.

For anyone who feels that they may lack the skills to provide meaningful feedback to colleagues there are various models that can be used which provide frameworks to help focus and structure feedback. One commonly used is known as Pendleton's Rules (Pendleton et al., 1984) and, while this is often used to guide feedback to trainees from their supervisors, the five stages are a good starting point to help underpin any feedback meeting. They are:

1. ask the person to whom you are giving feedback to highlight what areas of their practice they feel are going well, what their strengths are;
2. then the person providing the feedback tells their colleague what they feel is being done well and provides examples to highlight this;
3. next ask the person to tell you about any problems or concerns they might be having and how this might be impacting on their performance. Ask them how they might want to do things differently;
4. you then highlight your observations about any performance or behavioural issues that might be a cause for concern – you need to provide definitive examples and be specific;
5. the person receiving the feedback then identifies how they would like to change their performance or behaviour and what they might need in terms of support to do this.

There are many feedback models; Pendleton provides just one but is widely known and frequently used and, although not without criticism, is at the very least an aide to structuring a conversation that could be daunting for both parties. Using this framework requires you to consider the other person's perspective, to listen to their point of view and concerns and to allow them to find a solution and then to help them achieve it.

Take a moment to read the case study below.

Case study: Jenny

Jenny is a trainee nursing associate (TNA) and is a few weeks into a placement on an acute surgical ward. The environment has been challenging to Jenny as she has not worked in secondary care before, although she has got a lot of experience working in a community setting. Jenny has found many aspects of the placement outside her scope of practice and has tended to respond to this by avoiding the situation and instead finding areas that she is comfortable with and making herself busy with these.

Christine has been acting as Jenny's assessor in practice and has been both observing her and asking for feedback from the colleagues who have been working with Jenny. It is the mid-point, formative feedback meeting between student and assessor.

Christine makes the appointment to see Jenny and they agree to meet in the hospital library which has private tutorial rooms available. While Jenny is nervous, she has found Christine to be approachable and helpful. Christine starts by chatting about the ward and how it has been busy recently and asks Jenny some general questions about her time on the placement so far. The conversation turns to Jenny and Christine asks her to highlight what she most enjoys and what she feels that she has been achieving. Christine provides some examples of positive feedback that she has received and encourages Jenny to expand on what she has learned and done.

Christine then asks Jenny if there are any areas that she is finding a particular challenge or that she still feels unsure about. Christine is as equally encouraging as when highlighting Jenny's strengths; she underlines the point that the most effective practitioner is one that knows their own strengths but crucially their own limitations too. Jenny relaxes and explains that she has been feeling 'out of her depth' and has been less than proactive at addressing this. Christine agrees and says that she has been wondering if Jenny has been avoiding some of the more demanding or complex situations and has noticed that Jenny tends to stick to the things she is good at.

Christine asks Jenny to identify any recent events that she knows that she avoided – they discuss them and any specific reasons why they worried Jenny. Christine is non-judgemental and reassures Jenny that her actions are not unusual and are understandable; she asks her to identify what a different approach might look like and what support Jenny would need to take such an approach. Together they formulate a plan based on Jenny's suggestions and add this to a learning development form so that all those supporting Jenny can refer to it.

Activity 8.6   Reflection

Consider Jenny's case – as a TNA, is this an approach that you have encountered? If not – would this approach be helpful to you and, if this has not been your experience, perhaps using one of the models will help you in future when you have to feed back to colleagues. Our own experience does impact on our future practice, but you can decide to build on good examples or improve your skills if you feel you have not had such positive role models.

As this is a reflective activity no model answer has been provided at the end of the chapter.

It is important to recognise that providing feedback is a skill and to do so in a compassionate way means approaching that skill from a very committed perspective. One way to support this is to ensure that you are resourced and can reflect on your own strengths, challenges and even your own prejudices and preconceptions – we all have them! Clinical supervision is regular (although not necessarily frequent) and protected time for supported reflection on your clinical practise. The aim is to enable an employee to have the time and opportunity to really think about how they practise and to develop, understand and improve that practice with the meaningful and focused support of an appropriate facilitator. Formal supervision is a useful way to provide a focus for your reflective practice but also the permission and space in which to be reflective. Most organisations have a policy to support the idea of clinical supervision and it is a very good way to role model the importance of self-compassion and self-awareness.

Activity 8.7   Research

Access your organisation's human resources (HR) website – perhaps it is part of an intranet or, if you work for a private healthcare provider, it may be part of that organisation's main website. Search for their supervision policy and see what support and advice is contained within the policy. Were you aware of this policy's existence? Is there a policy? Are your colleagues aware of it or of the lack of it? Do any of your colleagues receive regular clinical or personal supervision within their working hours?

If you would like to access formal clinical supervision, why not have a discussion with your line manager; your annual performance development review (PDR) might be a good forum to raise this – you could be the catalyst that starts a culture of supervision in your workplace! ...

Each provider will have a different approach to supervision so no model answer will be provided for this activity. An anonymised supervision statement from an NHS trust which is freely and publicly available has been provided to act as an example.

The need to be open and honest

This next section is not supposed be a cautionary or negative counterpoint to the rest of this chapter – quite the opposite. It is, perhaps, a way of also acknowledging that compassionate cultures are not complacent or 'soft' cultures. The requirement to be open and honest and to exercise what is known as a 'duty of candour' is as much an aspect of compassionate support and intent as any other element. To ignore this does not assist or develop colleagues and does not provide the safe and patient-focused care that we all aspire to. The *Standards of Proficiency* (NMC, 2018c) highlight the need to be courageous and transparent by recognising and reporting anything that might result in poor care outcomes. In 2022 the NMC, jointly with the GMC, updated the guidance on the professional duty of candour. This guidance emphasises the importance of being open and honest, of telling people when things have gone wrong and especially the importance of apologising. Putting things right when mistakes occur is not simply about finding clinical solutions to errors, it is about acknowledging harm and hurt and being genuinely sorry that it has happened. Both elements are required for healing to occur.

Compassion might be the very skill that enables a healthcare professional to fulfil this duty of candour while also ensuring that they promote a no-blame culture where colleagues still feel supported and able to learn from mistakes rather than be condemned for them. A workplace where the idea of analysing mistakes, taking a team approach to any highlighted poor practices and emphasising compassion and care underpins any performance management activity will help set the overarching approach to supporting staff. West and Markiewicz (2016) describe how compassionate leadership promotes a culture of learning where it is safe to take reasonable risks to innovate and bring about positive changes. Practical approaches such as ensuring appropriate policies are in place and are known about and that meaningful and realistic risk assessments are consistently completed for both patients and staff are also important. The key message is that compassion and practicality, including the need to be open and honest, are not mutually exclusive but absolutely complementary.

Understanding the theory: duty of candour

There is a lot of anxiety related to 'duty of candour' as it can be construed as telling tales or giving people upsetting information. The NMC (2018a) makes it clear that this is a duty and not optional – there is a duty to be honest and open with patients and this needs to be part of an organisation's expectations and culture. Think back to the scenario about Tina, the nurse who made the drug error – mentioned earlier in this chapter and described in Chapter 4 – it would obviously be important to report the error immediately to relevant senior colleagues who could assess if the patient had been placed at any risk. If the mistake were to be covered up in any way, then this assessment might not happen and the patient could come to harm. Once the risk has been established then the patient would need to be informed of the error and of the steps taken to ensure their safety.

The importance of reflection and self-awareness: self-compassion as a leadership skill

This chapter has highlighted the importance of role modelling and of the benefits of accessing supervision to enable compassionate practice and leadership. This final part of the chapter aims to emphasise how important it is to be compassionate to yourself and, while this sounds straightforward, how this can be a significant challenge. There is a growing body of evidence that suggests that burnout and compassion fatigue is not caused by being too empathetic and compassionate to patients and colleagues as may have been a common perception. Instead, it is working in environments where there is no opportunity or expectation that this is how care should be provided – simply going to work to carry out tasks and to meet targets and to have no time to do anything but the most basic level of care undermines job satisfaction. While there were a range of factors that led to hundreds of untimely or totally avoidable patient deaths and injury at Mid-Staffordshire (as previously discussed in Chapter 7, see the Francis Report, 2013), lapses in compassion and compassion fatigue were highlighted as part of the problem in the report. So, lack of compassion has potentially disastrous consequences for patient care and safety; to address our own need for compassion is not an indulgence, it is a clinical and professional requirement.

Activity 8.8   Reflection

As with feedback, there are models to help you with your reflective practice. Please look up the following commonly used reflective models (there are others):

1. Gibbs, 1988
2. Johns, 1995
3. Schon, 1991

Spend some time thinking about a recent experience that you have had in practice that caused you to question either your own or a colleague's actions or a patient's response.

Now consider what happened applying the three frameworks above.

*   Did any of these frameworks help you make sense of the situation?
*   Which framework was easiest to use and made the most sense to you?
*   Did using a framework help you to reflect more easily and more productively – in short, was it better with a framework or not?

If it was easier and you found one model more suitable to your needs and understanding than another, it may be beneficial to add this to your practice in future as part of your 'self-compassion toolkit'.

As this is a reflective exercise, no model answer has been provided. There are some helpful websites to assist with this activity in the Useful websites section at the end of the chapter.

Reflective practice is not a new concept and has been the subject of books, articles and policies; it has resulted in frameworks and guidelines to help support and promote this practice. Suffice to say, in terms of self-compassion the ability to be reflective and to really prioritise this practice in your working life is a very positive step towards understanding your own strengths but also your own needs and challenges. To recognise when you might be at risk of becoming compassion fatigued, to understand how you are prioritising care provision and how you are supporting and giving feedback to colleagues takes commitment and self-awareness. If you are not able to access formal clinical supervision there is nothing stopping you from cultivating a reflective attitude; perhaps you could set up a group supervision meeting with your colleagues. What is there to stop you? Taking some focused time to reflect and discuss practice may well pay back the time taken many times over as challenges are identified, solutions found and support suggested. And if you and your colleagues feel more supported you are likely to be happier in your work and less likely to leave or become unwell with work-related stress.

Remember, leadership is everyone's responsibility so you can do this – you can be the role model.

Chapter summary

This chapter has described the importance of compassion and how compassionate leadership impacts on patient care. Compassion has been defined and this definition has then been used to underpin the link to leadership skills. Relevant policy that highlights compassion has been identified and related to professional values and attitudes. The activities and case studies that have been included aimed to help you establish how compassion can be demonstrated and what can happen when compassion is lacking. Ideas and theories that assist a practitioner to show their compassion have been suggested and include providing focused feedback, being open and honest and how important it is to be compassionate to yourself.

Activities: brief outline answers

Activity 8.2

- Empower colleagues – delegating tasks to colleagues when that task is within their capabilities allows them to feel involved and, if then followed up with feedback that highlights good practice, also empowered and effective.
- Don't engage in 'cliques' – make a concerted effort to involve and support everyone – reflect on times when you may have excluded a colleague or doubted their ability – did it make them more effective?
- Help a colleague – when it is possible, make a point of offering support to your wider team. If you have had a coffee break you could cover a colleague to enable them to take their break. And not just junior colleagues or peers – make sure your manager takes a break too – this sets a cultural expectation.
- Take time in each shift to 'step back' and reflect on where you are, what is happening and whether there needs to be a reconsideration or rebalancing. Sometimes five minutes spent considering what is going on can prevent mistakes or can identify if someone is struggling – addressing the situation early can save time in the long run and, more importantly, prevent mistakes and highlight compassionate intent.
- Consider the importance of promoting and encouraging your colleagues, if they take time to access education or training, if they have an ambition or idea – take time to consider how this will improve your environment and patient care. Be the positive and encouraging force in your team – you will benefit from a culture that promotes this when your turn comes to shine!

Activity 8.3

- Patients who perceive that their carers are focused on them and care about them are more likely to talk openly about their needs and provide relevant information on which to base a truly holistic assessment.
- Patients who feel 'heard' and 'seen' by those who are caring for them are more likely to feel as if their needs have been met and will not require further input.
- If patients believe you are motivated by compassion and kindness and that you care about them, they are more likely to comply with advice you provide, to be concordant.
- Patients who believe that you will help them and that you will care about their problems are more likely to ask for help in a timely way – you are therefore more able to deal with problems before they escalate and result in greater harm and greater need for resources.
- Patients who report that they received kind and compassionate care are more likely to recommend organisations or providers to others who will then be more likely to access timely intervention if they have health concerns.
- Patients who feel reassured and supported require fewer resources – research suggests that patients who report compassionate care require less analgesia, are discharged earlier, re-attend less frequently, have fewer complications of treatment and, ultimately, stay alive longer!

All the statements above are evidence-based – for further information read the books by Stephen Trzeciak and Anthony Mazzarelli, and Michael West listed in the Further reading section of this chapter.

Activity 8.4

- Do you feel sorry for Casey or, can you understand why some staff may have 'rolled their eyes'?

As far back as 1972 Felicity Stockwell wrote her ground-breaking book *The Unpopular Patient*, which detailed research indicating that nurses gave preferential care to favoured patients. Patients who frequently attend healthcare providers such as their GP or local hospital have been labelled as 'revolving door' patients and evidence suggest that they do not always receive the most compassionate care.

- Why do you think Casey starts to cry?

People, especially when feeling vulnerable, need to feel they matter, that they are important and have been acknowledged. Crying is a normal response when someone is kind and compassionate – this can be because they are given 'permission' to let their vulnerability and distress show; this is known as a cathartic response.

- What do you think will be the benefit to Casey, to the NA and to the ED because of the way the NA approached Casey?

As described in the research in the chapter, Casey is less likely to return to ED, benefitting both her and the department. As for the NA? He should feel justly proud of his intervention, a sense of achievement that he has helped a patient who is clearly suffering and job satisfaction that he can exercise compassionate practice.

Activity 8.7

Example of a trust policy on clinical supervision:

> Clinical supervision is 'regular, protected time for facilitated in-depth reflection on clinical practice. It aims to enable the supervisee to achieve, sustain and creatively develop a high quality of practice through the means of focused support and development ... whether they remain in clinical practice or move into management, research or education' Bond and Holland (1998: 12).

> Within [the anonymised] trust we are aiming to ensure that every registered practitioner has access to clinical supervision. We expect practitioners to receive a minimum of four hours clinical supervision per annum, although clinical areas differ, and you should be able to access as much clinical supervision as you feel is necessary.

> (Anonymised source)

Further reading

Trzeciak, S. and Mazzarelli, A. (2019) *Compassionomics: The Revolutionary Scientific Evidence That Caring Makes a Difference*. Florida: Studer.

This book contains a lot of information and evidence about the impact of compassion on patient care; the authors describe compassion as a 'science' that can be studied.

West, M.A. (2021) *Compassionate Leadership: Sustaining Wisdom, Humanity and Presence in Health and Social Care*. London: Swirling Leaf Press.

This book highlights how leadership specifically benefits from a compassionate focus and the power that compassion has to impact patient care and staff well-being.

Useful websites

www.kingsfund.org.uk/publications/what-is-compassionate-leadership

Follow this URL to the King's Fund pages that describe many aspects of compassionate leadership, including the behaviours that demonstrate this but also what can get in the way of being a compassionate leader.

www.nmc.org.uk/globalassets/sitedocuments/revalidation/reflective-practice-guidance.pdf

This web link will take you to the NMC site relating to the reflections needed by RNAs when they have to revalidate in order to remain on the NMC register. A useful reminder of the importance of reflection and why you need to be proficient in this skill.

www.rcn.org.uk/Professional-Development/Revalidation/Reflection-and-reflective-discussion

This link will take you to the RCN pages related to reflection and includes further links to several of the models mentioned in the activities in this chapter.

References

Affina Organisation Development (2022) *Affina Team Performance Inventory.* Available at: www.affinaod.com/wp-content/uploads/2022/04/ATPI_Sample-Team-A. pdf (accessed 23 June 2023).

Andrews, K.R. (1971) *The Concept of Corporate Strategy.* Homewood, IL: Irwin.

Atsalos, C. and Greenwood, J. (2001) The lived experience of clinical development unit (nursing) leadership in Western Sydney, Australia. *Journal of Advanced Nursing*, 34(3): 408–416.

Baillie, N. (2014) *NICE Quality Standards and Indicators.* London: NICE.

Ball, J., Maben, J., Murrells, T., Day, T. and Griffiths, P. (2015) *12-hour Shifts: Prevalence, Views and Impact.* National Nursing Research Unit, King's College London.

Banning, M. (2008) A review of clinical decision making: models and current research. *Journal of Clinical Nursing*, 17(2): 187–195.

Barr, J. and Dowding, L. (2019) *Leadership in Healthcare.* London: Sage.

Barrett, B. and Heale, R. (2021) Covid-19: reflections on its impact on nursing. *Evidence-based Nursing*, 24(4).

Bass, B.M. (1992) Assessing the charismatic leader. In M. Syrett and C. Hogg (eds.), *Frontiers of Leadership.* Oxford: Blackwell.

Bass, B.M. and Avolio, B.J. (1995) *The Multifactor Leadership Questionnaire: 5x Short Form.* Redwood City, CA: Mind Garden.

Bass, B.M. and Riggio, R.E. (2006) *Transformational Leadership.* London: Lawrence Erlbaum Associates.

Baverstock, A. and Finlay, F. (2019) Take a break: HALT – are you hungry, angry, late or tired? *Archives of Disease in Childhood. Education and Practice Edition*, 104(4): 200.

Beauchamp, T.L. and Childress, J.F. (2013) *Principles of Biomedical Ethics* (8th ed.). New York: Oxford University Press.

Beetham, H. (2017) Digital capabilities framework: an update. Jisc, 9 March. Available at: https://digitalcapability.jiscinvolve.org/wp/2017/03/09/digital-capabilities-framework-an-update/ (accessed 6 June 2023).

Belbin, R.M. (2000) *Beyond the Team* (1st ed.). London: Routledge. doi.org/10.4324/9780080500065.

Benjamin, A. (2008) Audit: how to do it in practice. *BMJ*, 336(7655): 1241–1245.

Benner, P. (2001[1984]) *From Novice to Expert: Excellence and Power in Clinical Nursing Practice.* London/Menlo Park, CA: Addison-Wesley.

Betts, L.R., Hill, R. and Gardner, S.E. (2019) 'There's not enough knowledge out there': examining older adults' perceptions of digital technology use and digital inclusion classes. *Journal of Applied Gerontology*, 38(8): 1147–1166.

British Medical Association (BMA) (2022) *BMA Covid Review 3: Delivery of Healthcare during the Pandemic*. Available at: bma-covid-review-report-3-june-2022.pdf (accessed 23 June 2023).

Brookes, N. (2021) How to undertake effective record-keeping and documentation. *Nursing Standard*. doi:10.7748/ns.2021.e11700.

Brown, D. and Hilson, N. (2014) What to do to prepare for a CQC inspection. *Practice Nursing*, 25(8). doi.org/10.12968/pnur.2014.25.8.401.

Brown, J., Pope, N., Bosco, A., Mason, J. and Morgan, A. (2020) Issues affecting nurses' capability to use digital technology at work: an integrative review. *Journal of Clinical Nursing*, 29(15–16): 2801–2819.

Buchanan, D.A. and Huczynski, A. (2019) *Organisational Behaviour* (10th ed.). London: Pearson.

Burns, C. and West, M.A. (2003) Individual, climate, and group interaction processes as predictors of work team innovation. *Small Group Research*, 26: 106–117.

Burns, J.M. (1978) *Leadership*. New York: Harper & Row.

Callaghan, L. (2007) Advanced nursing practice: an idea whose time has come. *Journal of Clinical Nursing*, 17(2): 205–213.

Cambridge English Dictionary (2022) Interdisciplinary. *Cambridge English Dictionary*. Available at: https://dictionary.cambridge.org/dictionary/english/interdisciplinary (accessed 24 July 2022).

Care Opinion (2022) *About Care Opinion*. Available at: www.careopinion.org.uk/info/about (accessed 14 July 2023).

Care Quality Commission (CQC) (2022) *What does good care look like?* Available at: www.cqc.org.uk/care-services/what-expect-good-care-service (accessed 14 July 2023).

CQC (2023) *About Us*. Available at: www.cqc.org.uk/about-us (accessed 14 July 2023).

Chambers, R. and Wakely, G. (2005) *Clinical Audit in Primary Care: Demonstrating Quality Outcomes*. Oxford: Radcliffe.

Christian, M.D. (2019) Triage. *Critical Care Clinics*, 35(4): 575–589. doi: 10.1016/j.ccc.2019.06.009. Epub 2019 Jul 27. PMID: 31445606; PMCID: PMC7127292

Clark, C. (2021) *Why Nurses Eat Their Young and How to Stop This Damaging Practice*. American Association of Post-Acute Care Nursing. Available at: www.aapacn.org/article/why-nurses-eat-their-young-and-how-to-stop-this-damaging-practice/ (accessed 23 June 2023).

Commonwealth Fund (2021) *Mirror, Mirror 2021: Reflecting Poorly. Health Care in the US Compared to Other High-Income Countries*. doi.org/10.26099/01dv-h208.

Covey, S.R. (1989) *The 7 Habits of Highly Effective People*. London: Simon & Schuster.

Crawford, J. and Daniels, M.K. (2014) Follow the leader: how does 'followership' influence nurse burnout? *Nursing Management*, 45(8): 30–37.

Cummings, J. and Bennett, V. (2012) *Compassion in Practice: Nursing, Midwifery and Care Staff. Our Vision and Strategy.* Department of Health. Available at: www.england.nhs.uk/wp-content/uploads/2012/12/compassion-in-practice.pdf (accessed 23 June 2023).

Data Protection Act 2018, c. 12. Available at: www.legislation.gov.uk/ukpga/2018/12/ Davey, M. (2019) My trainee nursing associate role. *British Journal of Healthcare Assistants,* 13(3): 131–133.

Deakin, M. (2022) NHS workforce shortages and staff burnout are taking a toll. *British Medical Journal,* 377: o945.

Department of Health (DoH) (1997) *The New NHS: Modern. Dependable.* London: HMSO.

DoH (2012) *Transforming Care: A National Response to Winterbourne View Hospital.* London: DoH.

DoH (2022) *Clinical Governance.* Available at: www.gov.uk/government/publications/newborn-hearing-screening-programme-nhsp-operational-guidance/4-clinical-governance (accessed 23 June 2023).

Department of Health and Social Care (DoHSC) (2010) *Liberating the NHS.* Available at: www.gov.uk/government/publications/liberating-the-nhs-white-paper (accessed 23 June 2023).

DoHSC (2021) *The NHS Constitution for England.* Available at: www.gov.uk/government/publications/the-nhs-constitution-for-england (accessed 23 June 2023).

Dixon, N. and Pearce, M. (2011) *Guide to Ensuring Data Quality in Clinical Audits.* London: Healthcare Quality Improvement Partnership.

Doyle, C., Lennox, L. and Bell, D. (2013) A systematic review of evidence on the links between patient experience and clinical safety and effectiveness. *BMJ Open,* 3: e001570. doi:10.1136/bmjopen-2012-001570.

Drucker, P.F. (2007) *The Practice of Management* (Classic Drucker Collection edition). Oxford: Butterworth-Heinemann.

Dyer, J.G. and McGuinness, T.M. (1996) Resilience: analysis of the concept. *Archives of Psychiatric Nursing,* 10: 276–282.

Edwards, K., Jones, R.B., Shenton, D., Page, T., Maramba, I., Warren, A., Fraser, F., Križaj, T., Coombe, T., Cowls, H. and Chatterjee, A. (2021) The use of smart speakers in care home residents: implementation study. *Journal of Medical Internet Research,* 23(12): e26767.

Elliott, M. (2021) 'The global elements of vital signs' assessment: a guide for clinical practice. *British Journal of Nursing.* Available at: www.britishjournalofnursing.com/content/clinical/the-global-elements-of-vital-signs-assessment-a-guide-for-clinical-practice (accessed 23 June 2023).

Ellis, P. (2018) *Leadership, Management and Team Working in Nursing.* London: Sage.

Ellis, P. (2022) *Leadership, Management and Team Working in Nursing* (4th ed.). London: Sage.

Endsley, M.R. (1995) Toward a theory of situational awareness in dynamic systems. *Human Factors,* 37: 32–64. doi:10.1518/001872095779049543.

Flin, R., O'Connor, P. and Crichton, M. (2008) *Safety at the Sharp End: A Guide to Non-Technical Skills*. London: Ashgate.

Francis, R. (2013) *Report of the Mid Staffordshire NHS Foundation Trust Public Inquiry*. London: HMSO. Available at: www.gov.uk/government/publications/report-of-the-mid-staffordshire-nhs-foundation-trust-public-inquiry (accessed 23 June 2023).

Gage, W. (2016) Role of the nurse in managing complaints in their clinical area. *Nursing Standard*, 30. doi: 10.7748/ns.30.32.51.s44.

Gawande, A.A., Zinner, M.J., Stuudert, D.M. and Brenna, T.A. (2003) Analysis of errors reported by surgeons at three teaching hospitals. *Surgery*, 133(6): 614–621.

Gibbs, G. (1988) *Learning by Doing: A Guide to Teaching and Learning Methods*. Oxford: Oxford Polytechnic, Further Education Unit.

Gilbert, P. (2017) Compassion: definitions and controversies. In P. Gilbert (ed.), *Compassion: Concepts, Research and Applications*. London: Routledge. pp. 3–15.

Gillespie, G.L., Grubb, P.L., Brown, K., Boesch, M.C. and Ulrich, D. (2017) 'Nurses Eat Their Young': a novel bullying educational program for student nurses. *Journal of Nursing Education and Practice*, 7(7): 11–21.

Goleman, D. (1995) *Emotional Intelligence: Why It Can Matter More Than IQ*. New York: Bantam.

Goleman, D. (1998) *Working with Emotional Intelligence*. New York: Bantam.

Goleman, D. (2000) Leadership that gets results. *Harvard Business Review*, 78: 78–90.

Gopee, N. (2010) *Practice Teaching in Healthcare*. London: Sage. doi.org/10.4135/9781446251560.

Gopee, N. (2022) *Leading and Managing Healthcare*. London: Sage.

Gopee, N. and Galloway, J. (2017) *Leadership and Management in Healthcare* (3rd ed.). London: Sage.

Gordon, L.J., Rees, C.E., Ker, J.S. and Jennifer Cleland, J. (2015) Dimensions, discourses and differences: trainees conceptualising health care leadership and followership. *Medical Education*, 49: 1248–1262. doi: 10.1111/medu.12832.

Gorgich, E.A.C., Barfroshan, S., Ghoreishi, G. and Yaghoobi, M. (2016) Investigating the causes of medication errors and strategies to prevention of them from nurses and nursing student viewpoint. *Global Journal of Health Science*, 8(8): 320–327.

Griffith, R. (2018) District nurses must guard against inappropriately accessing patient records. *British Journal of Community Nursing*, 23(7): 355.

Griffith, R. and Tengnah, C. (2017) *Law and Professional Issues in Nursing*. London: Sage.

Grossman, S. and Valiga, T. (2012) *The New Leadership Challenge: Creating the Future of Nursing* (4th ed.). Philadelphia: FA Davis.

Hamm, R.M. (1988) Clinical intuition and clinical analysis: expertise and the cognitive continuum. In J. Dowie and A. Elstein (eds.), *Professional Judgement: A Reader in Clinical Decision Making*. Cambridge: Cambridge University Press.

Hammond, K.R. (1981) *Principles of Organization in Intuitive and Analytical Cognition* (Report 231). Center for Research on Judgement and Policy, University of Colorado, Boulder, CO.

Harmer, M. (2010) *Independent Review on the care given to Mrs Elaine Bromiley on 29 March 2005.* Available at: https://emcrit.org/wp-content/uploads/ElaineBromiley AnonymousReport.pdf (accessed 21 June 2022).

Health and Safety Executive (HSE) (2021) *Introduction to Human Factors.* Available at: www.hse.gov.uk/humanfactors/introduction.htm (accessed 23 June 2023).

Health Education England (HEE) (2015) *Raising the Bar: Shape of Caring: A Review of the Future Education and Training of Registered Nurses and Care Assistants.* Available at: https://hee.nhs.uk/sites/default/files/documents/2348-Shape-of-caring-review-FINAL.pdf (accessed 18 September 2022).

HEE (2017) *A Health and Care Digital Capabilities Framework.* London: HEE.

HEE (2018) *Maximising Leadership Learning in the Pre-Registration Healthcare Curricula Model and Guidelines for Healthcare Education Providers.* Available at: www.hee.nhs.uk/sites/default/files/documents/Guidelines%20-%20Maximising%20 Leadership%20in%20the%20Pre-reg%20Healthcare%20Curricula%20%282018%29.pdf (accessed 23 June 2023).

HEE (2019a) *The Topol Review: Preparing the Healthcare Workforce to Deliver the Digital Future.* London: HEE.

HEE (2019b) *Why Employ a Nursing Associate? Benefits for Health and Care Employers.* London: HEE.

Healthcare Improvement Scotland (HIS) (2020) *Prevention and Management of Pressure Ulcers.* Edinburgh: HIS.

Hersey, P., Blachard, K. and Johnson, D.E. (1996) *Management of Organizational Behaviour: Utilizing Human Resources* (7th ed.). Englewood Cliffs, NJ: Prentice-Hall.

Hersey, P., Blanchard, K.H. and Johnson, D.E. (2001) *Management of Organizational Behaviour.* Escondido, CA: Centre for Leadership Studies.

Hojat, M., Bianco, J.A., Mann, D., Massello, D. and Calabrese, L.H. (2014) Overlap between empathy, teamwork and integrative approach to patient care. *Medical Teacher,* 37: 755–758.

Institute for Healthcare Improvement (IHI) (2016) *Plan–Do–Study–Act (PDSA) Worksheet.* Boston, MA: IHI.

Jack, K., Bianchi, M., Dilar Pereira Costa, R., Grinberg, K., Harnett, G., Luiking, M., Nilsson, S. and Scammell, J.M.E. (2022) Clinical leadership in nursing students: a concept analysis. *Nurse Education Today,* 108: 105173, ISSN 0260-6917. doi. org/10.1016/j.nedt.2021.105173.

Jaffe, A. and Jung, C. (1965) *Memories, Dreams, Reflections.* New York: Random House.

Johns, C. (1995) Framing learning through reflection within Carper's fundamental ways of knowing in nursing. *Journal of Advanced Nursing,* 22(2): 226–234.

Kahneman, D. (2013) *Thinking Fast and Slow*. New York: Farrar, Straus and Giroux.

Kelley, R. (1992) *The Power of Followership*. New York: Doubleday.

Kessler, I., Steils, N., Harris, J., Manthorpe, J. and Moriarty, J. (2021) *NHS Trust Survey 2020 on the Nursing Associate Role: Emerging Findings*. NIHR Policy Research Unit in Health and Social Care Workforce, Policy Institute, King's College London.

King, R., Robertson, S., Senek, M., Taylor, B., Ryan, T., Wood, E. and Tod, A. (2021) Impact of Covid-19 on the work, training and wellbeing experiences of nursing associates in England: A cross sectional survey. *Nursing Open*, 9: 1822–1831.

King's Fund (2012) *Leadership and Engagement for Improvement in the NHS: Together We Can*. London: King's Fund.

King's Fund (2022) *Overview of the Health and Social Care Workforce*. Available at: www.kingsfund.org.uk/projects/time-think-differently/trends-workforce-overview (accessed 23 June 2023).

Kotera, Y., Taylor, E., Fido, D., Williams, D. and Mccaie, F.T. (2021) Motivation of UK graduate students in education: self-compassion moderates pathway from extrinsic motivation to intrinsic motivation. *Current Psychology*, 42: 10163–10176. doi.org/10.1007/s12144-021-02301-6.

Kotter, J. (1990) *A Force for Change: How Leadership Differs from Management*. New York Free Press.

Kotter, J.P. (1995) Leading change: why transformation efforts fail. *Harvard Business Review*, 73: 259–267.

Kottner, J., Hahnel, E., Lichterfeld-Kottner, A., Blume-Peytavi, U. and Büscher, A. (2018) Measuring the quality of pressure ulcer prevention: a systematic mapping review of quality indicators. *International Wound Journal*, 15(2): 218–224. doi.org/10.1111/iwj.12854.

Kouzes, J.M. and Posner, B.Z. (2011) Leadership begins with an inner journey. *Leader to Leader*, 60: 22–27.

Kouzes, J.M. and Posner, B.Z. (2013) *The Student Leadership Challenge*. San Francisco: Wiley.

Leung, C., Lucas, A., Brindley, P., Anderson, S., Park, J., Vergis, A. and Gillman, L.M. (2018) Followership: a review of the literature in healthcare and beyond. *Journal of Critical Care*, 46: 99–104. ISSN 0883-9441. doi.org/10.1016/j.jcrc.2018.05.001.

Lewin, K. (1951) *Field Theory in Social Science*. London: Harper Row.

Lewin, K., Lippett, R. and White, R.K. (1939) Patterns of aggressive behaviour in experimentally created social climates. *Journal of Social Psychology*, 10.

Loveday, H.P., Wilson, J.A., Pratt, R.J., Golsorkhi, M., Tingle, A., Bak, A., Browne, J., Prieto, J. and Wilcox, M. (2014) *Pressure Ulcers: Prevention in Adults. Clinical Audit Report*. NICE. Available at: www.nice.org.uk/guidance/cg179/resources/clinical-audit-tool-pressure-ulcers-prevention-in-adults-excel-248685517 (accessed 23 June 2023).

Lucas, G., Brook, J., Thomas, T., Daniel, D., Ahmet, L. and Salmon, D. (2021) Healthcare professionals' views of a new second-level nursing associate role: a qualitative study exploring early implementation in an acute setting. *Journal of Clinical Nursing*, 30: 1312–1324. doi-org.plymouth.idm.oclc.org/10.1111/jocn.15675.

Luft, J. and Ingham, H. (1955) *The Johari Window: A Graphic Model for Interpersonal Relations*. Los Angeles: University of California, Western Training Lab.

Lyell, D., Magrabi, F., Raban, M.Z., Pont, L.G., Baysari, M.T. and Day, R.O. (2017) Automation bias in electronic prescribing. *BMC Medical Informatics and Decision Making*, 17(1): 1–7. doi:10.1186/s12911-017-0529-y.

Malenfant, S., Jaggi, P., Hayden, K.A. and Sinclair, S. (2022) Compassion in healthcare: an updated scoping review of the literature. *BMC Palliative Care*, 21: 80

Marquis, B.L. and Huston, C.J. (2012) *Leadership and Management Tools for the New Nurse: A Case Study Approach*. Philadelphia: Lippincott Williams & Wilkins.

Marquis, B.L. and Huston, C.L. (2017) *Leadership Roles and Management Functions in Nursing Theory and Application* (9th international ed.). Philadelphia: Wolters Kluwer.

McCance, T. and McCormack, B. (2016) *Person-Centred Practice in Nursing and Health Care: Theory and Practice* (2nd ed.). West Sussex: Wiley Blackwell.

McKinney, L. and Morris, P.A. (2010) Examining an evolution: a case study of organizational change accompanying the community college baccalaureate. *Community College Review*, 37(3): 187–208.

McKinnon, J. (2017) In their shoes: an ontological perspective on empathy in nursing practice. *Journal of Clinical Nursing*, 27: 3882–3889.

Meires, J. (2018) The essentials: using emotional intelligence to curtail bullying in the workplace. *Urologic Nursing*, 38: 150.

Melin-Johansson, C., Palmqvist, R. and Ronnberg, L. (2017) Clinical intuition in the nursing process and decision-making: a mixed-studies review. *Journal of Clinical Nursing*, 26: 3936–3949. doi.org/10.1111/jocn.13814.

Mind (2023) *Independent Review Launched at the Edenfield Centre*. Available at: www.mind.org.uk/news-campaigns/news/independent-review-launched-at-the-edenfield-centre/ (accessed 14 July 2023).

Mitchell, G. (2021) Nursing leaders denounce Covid-19 deniers. *Nursing Times*. Available at: www.nursingtimes.net/news/coronavirus/nursing-leaders-denounce-covid-19-deniers-08-01-2021/ (accessed 31 January 2023).

Mok, H. and Stevens, P. (2005) Models of decision making. In M. Raynor, J. Marshall and A. Sullivan (eds.), *Decision Making in Midwifery Practice*. Edinburgh: Churchill Livingstone–Elsevier. pp. 53–66.

Mumma, C.M. and Nelson, A. (2008) Theory and practice models for rehabilitation nursing. In S.P. Hoeman, *Rehabilitation Nursing: Process, Application and Outcomes* (4th edn). St Louis, MI: Mosby.

Murphy, M., Scott, L.J., Salisbury, C., Turner, A., Scott, A., Denholm, R., Lewis, R., Iyer, G., Macleod, J. and Horwood, J. (2021) Implementation of remote consulting in UK primary care following the Covid-19 pandemic: a mixed-methods longitudinal study. *British Journal of General Practice*, 71(704): e166–e177. doi: 10.3399/BJGP.2020.0948. PMID: 33558332; PMCID: PMC7909923

Murray, M., Sundin, D. and Cope, V. (2019) Benner's model and Duchscher's theory: providing the framework for understanding new graduate nurses' transition to practice. *Nurse Education in Practice*, 34: 199–203.

Nandasoma, U. (2019) Managing patient complaints. *MDU Journal*. Available at: https://mdujournal.themdu.com/issue-archive/ (accessed 23 June 2023).

National Audit Office (2018) *Investigation: WannaCry Cyber Attack and the NHS*. London: Department of Health.

National Cyber Security Centre (2022) *Phishing Attacks: Defending Your Organisation*. NCSC: United Kingdom.

National Data Guardian (2020) *The Caldicott Principles*. Available at: www.gov.uk/government/publications/the-caldicott-principles (accessed 12 July 2023).

National Guardian's Office (2021) *Developing Freedom to Speak Up Champion and Ambassador Networks: Guidance for Freedom to Speak Up Guardians*. London: National Guardian's Office.

National Health Service (NHS) (2018) *NHS Staff Survey: National Results*. www.nhsstaffsurveys.com/results/national-results/ (accessed 23 June 2023).

National Health Service (NHS) (2021) *NHS Staff Survey: National Results*. www.nhsstaffsurveys.com/results/national-results/ (accessed 4 March 2023).

National Institute for Health and Care Excellence (NICE) (2002) *Principles for Best Practice in Clinical Audit*. London: NICE.

Neves, A.L., Freise, L., Larange, L., Carter, A., Darzi, A., and Mayer, E. (2020) Impact of providing patient access to electronic health records on quality and safety of care: a systematic review and meta-analysis. *BMJ Quality and Safety*, 29: 019–1032

NICE (2012) *Healthcare-associated Infections: Prevention and Control in Primary and Community Care: Clinical Guideline* [CG139]. London: NICE.

NICE (2013) *Mental Wellbeing of Older People in Care Homes: Quality Standard* [QS50]. London: NICE.

NICE (2014) *Clinical Audit Tool: Pressure Ulcer Prevention in Adults*. Available at: www.nice.org.uk/guidance/cg179/resources (accessed 14 July 2023).

NICE (2015) *Pressure Ulcers: Quality Standard* [QS89]. London: NICE.

NICE (2016) *Recent-onset Chest Pain of Suspected Cardiac Origin: Assessment and Diagnosis: Clinical Guidelines* [CG95]. London: NICE.

NICE (2018) *Evidence Standards Framework for Digital Health Technologies: Corporate Document* [ECD7]. London: NICE.

NICE (2019) *Patient Experience in Adult NHS Services: Quality Standard* [QS15]. London: NICE.

National Institute for Health and Care Research (NIHR) (2022) *Health Information: Are You Getting Your Message Across?* Available at: https://evidence.nihr.ac.uk/collection/health-information-are-you-getting-your-message-across/ (accessed 12 July 2023).

National Quality Board (2013) *Quality in the New Health System: Maintaining and Improving Quality from April 2013*. London: DoHSC.

Neumann, T.A. (2010) Delegation: better safe than sorry. *AAOHN Journal*, 58(8): 321–322.

NHS Digital (2021a) *Around Half of People in England Now Have Access to Digital Healthcare.* Available at: https://digital.nhs.uk/news/2021/around-half-of-people-in-england-now-have-access-to-digital-healthcare (accessed 23 June 2023).

NHS Digital (2021b) *Guidance on Phishing Emails.* Available at: https://digital.nhs.uk/cyber-and-data-security/guidance-and-assurance/guidance-on-phishing-emails (accessed 23 June 2023).

NHS Digital (2021c) *NHS Workforce Statistics: January 2021 (Including Selected Provisional Statistics for February 2021).* Available at: https://digital.nhs.uk/data-and-information/publications/statistical/nhs-workforce-statistics/january-2021 (accessed 23 June 2023).

NHS Digital (2022) *NHS Workforce Statistics: May 2022 (Including Selected Provisional Statistics for June 2022).* Available at: https://digital.nhs.uk/data-and-information/publications/statistical/nhs-workforce-statistics/may-2022 (accessed 23 June 2023).

NHS England (2014) *MDT Development: Working Toward an Effective Multidisciplinary/Multiagency Team.* Available at: www.england.nhs.uk/wp-content/uploads/2015/01/mdt-dev-guid-flat-fin.pdf (accessed 24 July 2022).

NHS England (2015) *Guide for General Practice Staff on Reporting Patient Safety Incidents to the National Reporting and Learning System.* London: NHS England.

NHS England (2017) *Next Steps on the Five Year Forward View.* London: NHS England.

NHS England (2019) *The NHS Long Term Plan.* Available at: www.england.nhs.uk/long-term-plan (accessed 23 June 2023).

NHS England (2020) *Friends and Family Test.* Available at: www.england.nhs.uk/fft/ (accessed 14 July 2023).

NHS England (2021) *Records Management Code of Practice.* London: NHS Transformation Directorate.

NHS England (2022a) *Civility and Respect Toolkit.* Available at: www.england.nhs.uk/supporting-our-nhs-people/health-and-wellbeing-programmes/civility-and-respect/ (accessed 23 June 2023).

NHS England (2022b) *Coronavirus (Covid-19).* Available at: www.nhs.uk/conditions/covid-19/covid-19-symptoms-and-what-to-do/ (accessed 23 June 2023).

NHS England (2023) *Commissioning for Quality and Innovation (CQUIN): 2023/24.* London: NHS England (accessed 12 February 2023).

NHS England (n.d.a) *Governance, Patient Safety and Quality.* Available at: www.england.nhs.uk/mat-transformation/matrons-handbook/governance-patient-safety-and-quality/ (accessed 20 September 2022).

NHS England (n.d.b) *New Ways to Work in General Practice: New Types of Consultation.* Available at: www.england.nhs.uk/wp-content/uploads/2017/10/e-consult.pdf (accessed 23 June 2023).

NHS England and NHS Improvement (2021) *Building Strong Integrated Care Systems Everywhere.* Available at: www.england.nhs.uk/wp-content/uploads/2021/06/B0664-ics-clinical-and-care-professional-leadership.pdf (accessed 23 June 2023).

NHS Improvement (2018) *The Learning Disability Improvement Standards for NHS Trusts*. Available at: v1.17_Improvement_Standards_added_note.pdf (england.nhs.uk)

NHS Improvement (2019) *The NHS Patient Safety Strategy: Safer Culture, Safer Systems, Safer Patients*. London: NHS England.

NHS Leadership Academy (2013) *Healthcare Leadership Model*. Available at: www.leadershipacademy.nhs.uk/wp-content/uploads/2014/10/NHSLeadership-LeadershipModel-colour.pdf (accessed 23 June 2023).

NHS Leadership Academy (2023) *Healthcare Leadership Model: The Nine Dimensions of Leadership Behaviour*. NHS Leadership Academy. Available at: www.leadershipacademy.nhs.uk/wp-content/uploads/dlm_uploads/2014/10/NHSLeadership-LeadershipModel-colour.pdf (accessed 23 June 2023).

NHS Scotland (2010) *Scottish Audit of Surgical Mortality Annual Report*. NHS Scotland.

NHS Staff survey results are available at: www.nhsstaffsurveys.com/ (accessed 23 June 2023).

Northouse, P.G. (2019) *Leadership: Theory and Practice*. Los Angeles: Sage.

Nuffield Trust (2022) *The NHS Workforce in Numbers: Facts on Staffing and Staff Shortages in England*. Available at: www.nuffieldtrust.org.uk/resource/the-nhs-workforce-in-numbers (accessed 23 June 2023).

Nursing and Midwifery Council (NMC) (2018a) *The Code: Professional Standards of Practice and Behaviour for Nurses, Midwives and Nursing Associates*. London: NMC.

NMC (2018b) *Delegation and Accountability: Supplementary Information to the NMC Code*. Available at: delegation-and-accountability-supplementary-information-to-the-nmc-code.pdf (accessed 23 June 2023).

NMC (2018c) *Standards of Proficiency for Nursing Associates*. London: NMC. www.nmc.org.uk/globalassets/sitedocuments/standards-of-proficiency/nursing-associates/nursing-associates-proficiency-standards.pdf (accessed 23 June 2023).

NMC (2019a) *Raising Concerns: Guidance for Nurses, Midwives and Nursing Associates*. London: NMC.

NMC (2019b) *Revalidation*. NMC: England. Available at: www.nmc.org.uk/globalassets/sitedocuments/revalidation/how-to-revalidate-booklet.pdf (accessed 11 July 2023).

NMC (2022) *Social Media Guidance*. London: NMC.

Oxford Learner's Dictionary (n.d.) Available at: www.oxfordlearnersdictionaries.com/definition/english (accessed 23 June 2023).

Panorama (2022) Undercover hospital: patients at risk. BBC. 22 September, 21:00.

Parliamentary and Health Service Ombudsman (PHSO) (2010) *Care and Compassion? Report of the Health Service Ombudsman on Ten Investigations into NHS Care of Older People*. Available at: www.ombudsman.org.uk/sites/default/files/2016-10/Care%20and%20Compassion.pdf (accessed 23 June 2023).

Patient Coalition for AI, Data and Digital Tech in Health (2022) Putting Patients First: Championing Good Practice in Combatting Digital Health Inequalities. Available at: www.patients-association.org.uk/Handlers/Download.ashx?IDMF=a0e5b459-388a-4825-86d6-77910882633c (accessed 23 June 2023).

Pavlou, P.A. (2003) Consumer acceptance of electronic commerce: integrating trust and risk with the technology acceptance model. *International Journal of Electronic Commerce*, 7(3): 101–134.

Peate, I. (2019) *Fundamentals of Assessment and Care Planning for Nurses*. Chichester: John Wiley.

Peek, N., Sujan, M. and Scott, P. (2020) Digital health and care in pandemic times: impact of Covid-19. *BMJ Health and Care Informatics*, 27. doi: 10.1136/bmjhci-2020-100166.

Pendleton, D., Schofield, T., Tate, P. and Havelock, P. (1984) *The Consultation: An Approach to Learning and Teaching*. Oxford: Oxford University Press.

Pierre, M., Hofinger, G. and Buerschaper, C. (2007) *Crisis management in Acute Care Settings: Human Factors and Team Psychology in a High Stakes Environment*. London: Springer.

Poorkavoos, M. (2016) *Compassionate Leadership: What is it and Why Do Organisations Need More of It*. Available at: www.roffeypark.ac.uk/knowledge-and-learning-resources-hub/compassionate-leadership/ (accessed 23 June 2023).

Pope, A. (1963) *The Poems of Alexander Pope* (a one-volume edition of the Twickenham text ed.), ed. by John Butt. New Haven, CT: Yale University Press. ISBN 0300003404. OCLC 855720858

Pretz, J.E. and Folse, V.N. (2010) Nursing experience and preference for intuition in decision making. *Journal of Clinical Nursing*, 20: 2878–2889.

Queen's Nursing Institute (QNI) (2022) *Nursing in the Digital Age 2023: Using Technology to Support Patients in the Home*. London: QNI.

Reason, J. (1991) *Human Error*. Cambridge: Cambridge University Press.

Redelmeier, D.A., Molin, J.-P. and Tibshirani, R.J. (1995) A randomised trial of compassionate care for the homeless in an emergency department. *The Lancet*, 345: 1131–1134.

Redfern, O., Griffiths, P., Maruotti, A., Saucedo, A., Smith, G. and the Missed Care Study Group (2019) The association between nurse staffing levels and the timeliness of vital signs monitoring: a retrospective observational study in the UK. *BMJ Open*, 9. doi: 10.1136/bmjopen-2019-032157.

Reid, J. and Bromiley, M. (2012) Clinical human factors: the need to speak up to improve patient safety. *Nursing Standard*, 26(35): 35–40.

Resuscitation Council (2021) *2021 Resuscitation Guidelines*. London: Resuscitation Council.

Robertson, S., King, R., Taylor, B., Laker, S., Wood, E., Senek, M., Tod, A. and Ryan, T. (2022) Development of the nursing associate role in community and primary care settings across England. *Primary Health Care*, 33(3). doi:10.7748/phc.2022.e1764.

Roland, D., Stilwell, P.A., Fortune, P., Alexander, J., Clark, S.J. and Kenny, S. (2021) Case for change: a standardised inpatient paediatric early warning system in England. *Archives of Disease in Childhood*, 106: 648–651. doi:10.1136/archdischild-2020-32046.

Royal College of Emergency Medicine (RCEM) (2017) *Initial Assessment of Emergency Department Patients*. Available at: SDDC_Intial_Assessment_Feb2017.pdf (rcem.ac.uk)

References

Royal College of Nursing (RCN) (2015) *The Case for Healthy Workplaces: Healthy Workplace, Healthy You.* London: RCN. Available at: www.rcn.org.uk/Professional-Development/publications/pub-004963 (accessed 23 June 2023).

RCN (2018) *Every Nurse an E-nurse: Insights from a Consultation on the Digital Future of Nursing.* London: RCN.

RCN (2022a) *Leadership Skills: How to Demonstrate Leadership Skills within Your Career.* Available at: www.rcn.org.uk/Professional-Development/Your-career/Nurse/Leadership-skills (accessed 23 June 2023).

RCN (2022b) *RCN Position on Clinical Supervision.* Available at: www.rcn.org.uk/About-us/Our-Influencing-work/Position-statements/rcn-position-on-clinical-supervision (accessed 23 June 2023).

RCN (2022c) *Where Compassion Exists Within a Clinical Team, the Team is More Effective, and Patient Safety and Satisfaction are Higher.* Available at: www.rcn.org.uk/congress/congress-events/compassion-fatigue (accessed 23 June 2023).

RCN (2023) *Duty of Care.* Available at: www.rcn.org.uk/Get-Help/RCN-advice/duty-of-care (accessed 23 June 2023).

RCN (n.d.) *Become a Nursing Associate.* Available at: www.rcn.org.uk/Professional-Development/Nursing-Support-Workers/Become-a-nursing-associate (accessed 11.July 2023).

Recio-Saucedo, A., Dall'Ora, C., Maruotti, A., Ball, J., Briggs, J., Meredith, P., Redfern, O.C., Kovacs, C., Prytherch, D., Smith, G.B. and Griffiths, P. (2018) What impact does nursing care left undone have on patient outcomes? Review of the literature. *Journal of Clinical Nursing*, 27(11–12): 2248–2259. https://doi.org/10.1111/jocn.14058.

Royal College of Physicians (RCP) (2017) *National Early Warning Score* (NEWS2). Available at: www.rcplondon.ac.uk/projects/outputs/national-early-warning-score-news-2 (accessed 23 June 2023).

Russell, N. (2021) Misinformation during Covid: how should nurse practitioners respond? *Journal for Nurse Practitioners*, 17(6). doi: 10.1016/j.nurpra.2021.03.013.

Scally, G. and Donaldson, L.J. (1998) Looking forward: clinical governance and the drive for quality improvement in the new NHS in England. *BMJ*, 317: 61–65.

Schon, D.A. (1991) *The Reflective Practitioner: How Professionals Think in Action.* Aldershot: Ashgate.

Serrat, O. (2017) *Knowledge Solutions.* Singapore: Springer. doi.org/10.1007/978-981-10-0983-9_37.

Shamir, B. (2007) From passive recipients to active co-producers: followers' roles in the leadership process. In B. Shamir, R. Pillai, M. Bligh and M. Uhl-Bien (eds.), *Follower-centered Perspectives on Leadership: A Tribute to the Memory of James R. Meindl.* Charlotte, NC: Information Age. pp. ix–xxxix.

Shaw, S. (2007) *Nursing Leadership.* Oxford: Blackwell.

Sinclair, S., Russell, L.B., Hack, T.F., Kondejewski, J. and Sawatzky, R. (2017) Measuring compassion in healthcare: a comprehensive and critical review. *Patient*, 10(4), 389–405.

Skills for Care (2018) *An Introduction to Workplace Culture: What is it and Why is it Important?* Leeds: Skills for Care.

Smajdor, A. (2013) Reification and compassion in medicine: a tale of two systems. *Clinical Ethics*, 8(4): 111–118.

Smith-Trudeau, P. (2017) Nursing leadership and followership reflections on the importance of followers. *Vermont Nurse Connection*, 20(1): 2–4. Available at: https://search.ebscohost.com/login.aspx?direct=true&AuthType=ip,url,shib&db=rzh&AN=120134268&site=ehost-live (accessed 6 September 2022).

Spencer, A. and Patel, S. (2019) Applying the Data Protection Act 2018 and General Data Protection Regulation principles in healthcare settings. *Nursing Management*. doi: 10.7748/nm.2019.e1806.

Staggers, N., Gassert, C.A. and Curran, C. (2002) A Delphi study to determine informatics competencies for nurses at four levels of practice. *Nursing Research*, 51(6): 383–390. Available at: https://doi.org/10.1097/00006199-200211000-00006 (accessed 4 January 2022).

Standing, T.S. and Anthony, M.K. (2008). Delegation: what it means to acute care nurses. *Applied Nursing Research*, 21(1): 8–14.

Stanley, D. (2017) *Clinical Leadership in Nursing and Healthcare: Values into Action* (2nd ed.). West Sussex: Wiley Blackwell.

Stockwell, F. (1972) *The Unpopular Patient*. London: RCN.

Stogdill, R.M. (1974) *Handbook of Leadership*. New York: Free Press.

Storey, J. and Holti, R. (2013) *Towards a New Model of Leadership for the NHS.* Available at: www.leadershipacademy.nhs.uk/wp-content/uploads/dlm_uploads/2014/10/Towards-a-New-Model-of-Leadership-2013.pdf (accessed 23 June 2023).

Strauss, C., Taylor, B.L., Gu, J., Baer, R., Jones, F. and Cavanagh, K. (2016) What is compassion and how can we measure it? A review of definitions and measures. *Clinical Psychology Review*, 47: 15–27.

Suhonen, R., Stolt, M., Habermann, M., Hjaltadottir, I., Vryonides, S., Tonnessen, S., Halvorsen, K., Harvey, C., Toffoli, L. and Scott, P.A. (2018) Ethical elements in priority setting in nursing care: A scoping review. RANCARE Consortium COST Action – CA 15208. *International Journal of Nursing Studies*, 88: 25–42. doi: 10.1016/j.ijnurstu.2018.08.006. Epub 2018 Aug 17. PMID: 30179768

Sullivan, E. and Garland, G. (2013) *Practical Leadership and Management in Healthcare: For Nurses and Allied Health Professionals* (2nd ed.). Harlow: Pearson Education.

Taylor, M.J., McNicholas, C., Nicolay, C., Darzi, A., Bell, D. and Reed, J.E. (2013) Systematic review of the application of the plan–do–study–act method to improve quality in healthcare. *BMJ Quality and Safety*. doi.org/10.1136/bmjqs-2013-001862.

The Lancet Rheumatology (2021) Going viral: misinformation in the time of Covid-19. *The Lancet*, 3(6). doi:10.1016/S2665-9913(21)00154-5.

Thompson, C. (1999) A conceptual treadmill: the need for 'middle ground' in clinical decision-making theory in nursing. *Journal of Advanced Nursing*, 30: 1222–1229.

Tomlinson, J. (2015) Using clinical supervision to improve the quality and safety of patient care: a response to Berwick and Francis. *BMC Medical Education,* 15(1003). doi: 10.1186/s12909-015-0324-3.

Triggle, N. (2017) *NHS cyber-attack: No 'second spike' but disruption continues.* Available at: www.bbc.co.uk/news/uk-39918426 (accessed 12 July 2023).

Trueland, J. (2021) Why delegation is important for nurse leaders. *Primary Health Care,* 31(5): 9–11. doi:10.7748/phc.31.5.9.s3.

Trzeciak, S. and Mazzarelli, A. (2019) *Compassionomics: The Revolutionary Scientific Evidence That Caring Makes a Difference.* Florida: Studer.

Tucker, B.A. and Russell, R.F. (2004) The influence of the transformational leader. *Journal of Leadership and Organizational Studies,* 10: 103–111.

Tuckman, B. (1965) Developmental sequence in small groups. *Psychological Bulletin,* 63(6): 384–399.

Tuckman, B.W. and Jensen, M.A.C. (1977) Stages of small-group development revisited. *Group and Organization Studies,* 2(4): 419–427.

Uhl-Bien, M., Riggio, R.E., Lowe, K.B. and Carsten, M.K. (2014). Followership theory: a review and research agenda. *Leadership Quarterly,* 25: 83–104.

UK GDPR (2018) Available at: www.legislation.gov.uk/ukpga/2018/12/contents/enacted (accessed 11 July 2023).

Vogel, S. and Flint, B. (2021) Compassionate leadership: how to support your team when fixing the problem seems impossible. *Nursing Management,* 4(1): 32–41. 10.7748/nm.2021.e1967 Epub 2021 Jan 26. PMID: 33496150

Warren, J. (2013) Informatics. In G. Sherwood and J. Barnsteiner (eds.), *Quality and Safety in Nursing: A Competency Approach to Improving Outcomes.* Hoboken, NJ: John Wiley & Sons. pp. 171–187.

Waterlow, J. (2005) *Pressure Ulcer Prevention Manual* (1st ed.). Taunton: Wound Care Society.

Webb, L. (2020) *Communication Skills in Nursing Practice.* London: Sage.

Weber, M. (1905) *The Protestant Ethic and Spirit of Capitalism: And Other Writings.* New York: Penguin.

West, M.A. (2021) *Compassionate Leadership: Sustaining Wisdom, Humanity and Presence in Health and Social Care.* London: Swirling Leaf Press.

West, M., Bailey, S. and Williams, E. (2020) *The Courage of Compassion Supporting Nurses and Midwives to Deliver High-Quality Care.* London: King's Fund. www.kingsfund.org.uk/publications/courage-compassion-supporting-nurses-midwives (accessed 24 June 2023).

West, M.A., Hirst, G., Richter, A. and Shipton, H. (2004) Twelve steps to heaven: successfully managing change through developing innovative teams. *European Journal of Work and Organizational Psychology,* 13(2): 269–299. doi: 10.1080/13594320444000092.

West, M.A. and Markiewicz, L. (2016) Effective team working in health care. In E. Ferlie, K. Montgomery and A. Reff Pederson (eds.), *The Oxford Handbook of Health Care Management*. Oxford University Press: Oxford.

Weydt, A. (2010) Developing delegation skills. *Journal of Issues in Nursing*, 15(2): 1H.

WhatsApp (2022) *WhatsApp Privacy Policy*. Available at: www.whatsapp.com/legal/privacy-policy-eea/?lang=en#privacy-policy-information-we-collect (accessed 24 June 2023).

White, D.E. and Grason, S. (2019) The importance of emotional intelligence in nursing care. *Journal of Comprehensive Nursing Research and Care*, 4: 152.

Whitmore, J. (2017) *Coaching for Performance: Principles and Practice of Coaching and Leadership* (5th ed.). London: Nicholas Brealey.

Wiens, J., Saria, S., Sendak, M., Ghassemi, M., Liu, V.X., Doshi-Velez, F. and Jung, K. (2019) Do no harm: a roadmap for responsible machine learning for health care. *Nature Medicine*, 25(9): 1337–1340. doi: 10.1038/s41591-019-0561-9.

World Health Organization (WHO) (2017) *Patient Safety: Making Health Care Safer*. Geneva: WHO.

WHO (2019) *Burn-out as an 'Occupational Phenomenon'*. Available at: www.who.int/mental_health/evidence/burn-out/en/ (accessed 24 June 2023).

WHO (2020a) *Maintaining Essential Health Services: Operational Guidance for the Covid-19 Context: Interim Guidance*, 1 June. Available at: https://apps.who.int/iris/handle/10665/332240 (accessed 24 June 2023).

WHO (2020b) *State of the World's Nursing: Investing in Education, Jobs, and Leadership*. Available at: https://apps.who.int/iris/handle/10665/331677 (accessed 24 June 2023).

Wong, B., Khurana, M., Smith, R., El-Omrani, O., Pold, A., Lofti, A., O'Leary, C. and Saminarsih, D. (2021) Harnessing the digital potential of the next generation of health professionals. *Human Resources for Health*, 19(50).

Index

Page numbers followed by *f* indicate figures; those followed by *t* indicate tables.